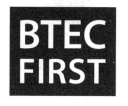

# BTEC FIRST

endorsed for
**BTEC**

## REVISE BTEC

# Sport

D1100126

Unit 1 Fitness for Sport and Exerci...

Unit 7 Anatomy and Physiology for S orts Performance

# REVISION GUIDE

Series Consultant: Harry Smith

Authors: Adam Gledhill and Sally Hillier

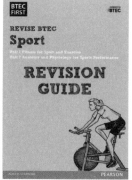

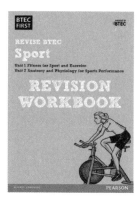

## THE REVISE BTEC SERIES

| | |
|---|---|
| BTEC First in Sport Revision Guide | 9781446906705 |
| BTEC First in Sport Revision Workbook | 9781446906712 |

This Revision Guide is designed to complement your classroom and home learning, and to help prepare you for the test. It does not include all the content and skills needed for the complete course. It is designed to work in combination with Pearson's main BTEC First series.

**To find out more visit:**
www.pearsonschools.co.uk/revise

ALWAYS LEARNING

**PEARSON**

Published by Pearson Education Limited, Edinburgh Gate, Harlow, Essex, CM20 2JE.

www.pearsonschoolsandfecolleges.co.uk

Copies of official specifications for all Pearson qualifications may be found on the website: www.edexcel.com

Text © Pearson Education Limited 2014
Typeset by Tech-Set Ltd, Gateshead
Original illustrations © Pearson Education Limited
Cover photo/illustration by Miriam Sturdee

The rights of Adam Gledhill and Sally Hillier to be identified as authors of this work has been asserted by them in accordance with the Copyright, Designs and Patents Act 1988.

First published 2014

17 16 15 14
10 9 8 7 6 5 4 3 2 1

**British Library Cataloguing in Publication Data**
A catalogue record for this book is available from the British Library

ISBN 978 1 4469 0670 5

Printed in Slovakia by Neografia

**Acknowledgements**
The publisher would like to thank the following for their kind permission to reproduce their photographs:
(Key: b-bottom; c-centre; l-left; r-right; t-top)

**Alamy Images:** Image Source Plus 16tr, Jonathan Larsen / Diadem Images 8t, 50b, Jonathan Larsen / Diadem Images 8t, 50b, Lucy Calder 8b, PhotoAlto sas 21b/I; **Corbis:** ARISTIDE ECONOMOPOULOS / Star Ledger 23, Kieran McManus / BPI 21b/iv, Peter Muller 21b/ii; **DK Images:** Gary Ombler 3b, Russell Sadur 27t; **Getty Images:** 4, 7b, 10b, 21b/iii, 53t, 53b, 54t, 54b, 55t, 61t, 62, 68, 69b, AFP 9, 20cl, 61b, 70t, 70c, BanksPhotos 41, Brian Pamphilon 20cr, Echo 51br, Mike Kemp 3t, Robert Cianflone 24, Steve Cole 26, Thomas Barwick 5b, XiXinXing 5t; **Science Photo Library Ltd:** ARNO MASSEE 30, GUSTOIMAGES 81; **Shutterstock.com:** Andi Berger 48, Galina Barskaya 29, helefty 65c, Maxisport 1, 55b, Michaelpuche 65t, Nicole Weiss 12, Olgysha 16bl, ostill 7r, 52b, Photobac 47, Photobac 47, Richard Paul Kane 65b, tankist276 52c, VOJTa Herout 6, zippy 67; **SuperStock:** Corbis 51bl; **Veer / Corbis:** Corepics 2, 51t, 52t, jcpjr 31, lightpoet 27b, MarFot 16bc, mindof 50t, moodboard Photography 28, 32, q-snap 10t, .shock 25, 70b, .shock 25, 70b, StepStock 7l, Sveter 16br, warrengoldswain 18, 27c, 66
All other images © Pearson Education

**Picture Research by:** Caitlin Swain
Every effort has been made to trace the copyright holders and we apologise in advance for any unintentional omissions. We would be pleased to insert the appropriate acknowledgement in any subsequent edition of this publication.

**A note from the publisher**

In order to ensure that this resource offers high-quality support for the associated BTEC qualification, it has been through a review process by the awarding body to confirm that it fully covers the teaching and learning content of the specification or part of a specification at which it is aimed, and demonstrates an appropriate balance between the development of subject skills, knowledge and understanding, in addition to preparation for assessment.

While the publishers have made every attempt to ensure that advice on the qualification and its assessment is accurate, the official specification and associated assessment guidance materials are the only authoritative source of information and should always be referred to for definitive guidance.

BTEC examiners have not contributed to any sections in this resource relevant to examination papers for which they have responsibility.

No material from an endorsed book will be used verbatim in any assessment set by BTEC.

Endorsement of a book does not mean that the book is required to achieve this BTEC qualification, nor does it mean that it is the only suitable material available to support the qualification, and any resource lists produced by the awarding body shall include this and other appropriate resources.

# Contents

This book covers the externally assessed units in the BTEC Level I/Level 2 First in Sport qualification.

Pearson publishes Sample Assessment Material and the Specification on its website. That is the official content, and this book should be used in conjunction with it. The questions in the *Now try this* sections have been written to help you practise every topic in the book. Remember: the real test questions may not look like this.

1-to-1 page match with the BTEC First in Sport Revision Workbook ISBN 978-1-446-90671-2

# Aerobic endurance

Aerobic endurance is one of the six components of physical fitness. It is important for any sustained physical activity.

Aerobic endurance is the ability of the CARDIORESPIRATORY SYSTEM to work efficiently, supplying NUTRIENTS and OXYGEN to working MUSCLES during sustained physical activity.

Activities that last for a long time require excellent aerobic endurance. Think of marathon running, long-distance swimming and triathlons.

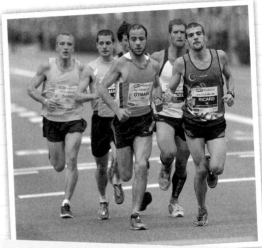

Marathon runners need excellent aerobic endurance to ensure that they can continue to run over a long distance.

## Physical fitness

There are six components of physical fitness:
- aerobic endurance
- muscular endurance
- flexibility
- speed
- muscular strength
- body composition.

You will learn about the other components in the following pages.

## Remember

AEROBIC means in the presence of oxygen.
ANAEROBIC means without oxygen.
Aerobic endurance is also known as cardiorespiratory fitness, cardiorespiratory endurance and aerobic fitness.

## The cardiorespiratory system

The cardiorespiratory system is made up of the cardiovascular system and the respiratory system.

The table to the right shows the components that make up each of these.

The cardiorespiratory system:
- uptakes oxygen from the air that you breathe in
- transports nutrients and oxygen around your body
- takes oxygen to working muscles
- removes waste products such as carbon dioxide from the body.

| Cardiovascular system | Respiratory system |
|---|---|
| Heart | Lungs |
| Blood | Airways |
| Blood vessels | |

## Worked example

There is only one mark available so think carefully about how much to write.

Give **one** reason why top-class sprinters do not require good aerobic endurance.
**(1 mark)**

Sprinters only work for very short periods of time so aerobic endurance is not a physical fitness requirement for them.

## Now try this

Explain **one** reason why aerobic endurance is important for an athlete competing in a triathlon.
**(2 marks)**

# Muscular endurance

Muscular endurance is one of the six components of physical fitness. It is important for sustained muscular activity involving light to moderate resistance.

Muscular endurance is the ability of the muscular system to work efficiently, where a muscle can continue contracting continuously against a light to moderate fixed resistance load.

In simple terms it is being able to use your muscles repeatedly without them getting tired.

## Voluntary muscles

Voluntary muscles are the muscles attached to your skeleton that help to produce movement.

For example, your abdominal muscles require good muscular endurance if you are going to complete a large number of sit-ups.

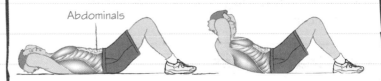
Abdominals

## Muscular endurance versus muscular strength

Muscular endurance and muscular strength are different.
Muscular endurance allows you to:
- work the muscles for a long time without getting tired
- work against light to moderate levels of resistance.

Muscular strength is about working for a shorter time against high levels of resistance. Weightlifters need muscular strength. You will revise muscular strength on page 5.

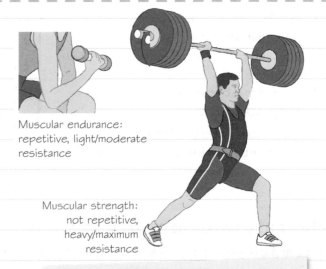
Muscular endurance: repetitive, light/moderate resistance

Muscular strength: not repetitive, heavy/maximum resistance

Don't confuse muscular endurance and muscular strength.

## Worked example

Look at the image of the rowing crew competing in a race.

Describe why these athletes need good muscular endurance for their event. **(2 marks)**

Rowers have excellent muscular endurance in their legs, back and arm muscles. They have to keep repeating the same movement against the resistance of the water for the duration of their race.

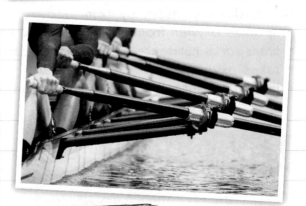

## Now try this

Make sure you refer to the length of the event.

Explain why a 1500 m swimmer requires good muscular endurance. **(2 marks)**

# Flexibility

Flexibility is one of the six components of physical fitness. Flexibility is important to ensure an adequate range of movement.

Flexibility can be defined as having an adequate range of motion in all joints of the body; the ability to move a joint fluidly through its complete range of movement.

## All-round flexibility

Some sports performers require good all-round flexibility. Gymnasts need high levels of flexibility in order to move, bend and flex their bodies around the different pieces of apparatus. Other sports performers might need flexibility in more specific joints. For example, hurdlers need good hip flexibility in order to achieve an accurate hurdling position.

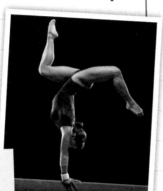

Gymnasts need high levels of flexibility.

## Stretching to improve flexibility

You can improve your flexibility by doing STRETCHING exercises. Stretching can help to make muscles more elastic so that your joints can move fluidly through their complete range of movement.

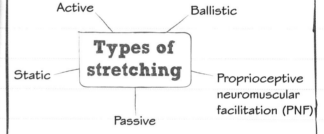

Active        Ballistic

**Types of stretching**

Static

Proprioceptive neuromuscular facilitation (PNF)

Passive

You will learn more about these types of stretches on pages 25 and 27.

## Worked example

The image shows a golfer preparing to swing.

Explain **one** reason why shoulder flexibility is important for this performer.                    **(2 marks)**

Having good shoulder flexibility allows the golfer to increase the range of motion in her swing so that more power can be applied to the ball to make it travel further.

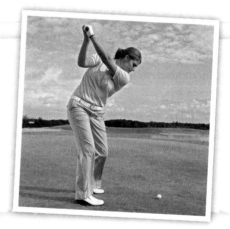

## Now try this

Flexibility is important in all sporting activities.

Complete the table below to show how flexibility would be used by each performer.                    **(3 marks)**

| Performer | How is flexibility used in their activity? |
|---|---|
| A figure skater during their routine | |
| A tennis player when hitting the ball | |
| A hurdler when clearing the hurdle | |

# Speed

Speed is one of the six components of physical fitness. Some sports are all about speed, such as sprinting, and many others involve speed combined with other components of physical fitness. Speed can be defined as: DISTANCE TRAVELLED DIVIDED BY TIME TAKEN. There are three types of speed.

 **Accelerative speed**

After sprinting for approximately 30 m, a sports performer will have accelerated to his or her top speed. In gymnastics, the vault run-up is approximately 25 m long, so the gymnast is almost at top speed when they reach it, increasing the height and distance of their vault.

## Calculating speed

Speed is measured in metres per second (m/s).

To work out how fast someone travelled you need to use the following formula:

$$\frac{\text{DISTANCE TRAVELLED}}{\text{TIME TAKEN}} = \text{SPEED (m/s)}$$

For example, if you run 100 m in 14 seconds, your speed would be calculated as follows:

$$\frac{100}{14} = 7.14 \text{ m/s}$$

 **Pure speed**

Some events, like sprints up to 60 m, are all about speed: the event is won by achieving the quickest time. The faster an athlete runs, the greater his or her speed.

 **Speed endurance**

Speed endurance is an athlete's ability to sustain maximum, or near maximum, episodes of speed over a prolonged period of time with short periods of recovery.

Footballers require good speed endurance – they spend lots of time chasing, moving and passing the ball but get periods of rest when the ball is not in their area of the pitch. Footballers can use speed to beat an opponent to a loose ball.

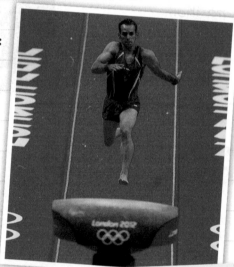

The vault run-up takes advantage of accelerative speed.

## Worked example

Don't forget to state the type of speed and then say why it is important.

There are three types of speed: accelerative speed, pure speed and speed endurance.

> Explain which type of speed is most important to a long jumper.   **(2 marks)**

> Accelerative speed is most important because a long jumper needs to be travelling at maximum speed at take-off to maximise the length of the jump.

Don't forget to show your workings.

## Now try this

An athlete runs 200 m in 24.5 seconds.

> Calculate the athlete's average speed over this distance.   **(2 marks)**

# Muscular strength

Muscular strength is one of the six components of physical fitness and is needed for activities that require force.

Muscular strength is the maximum force – measured in kilograms (kg) or newtons (n) – that can be generated by a muscle or group of muscles. Muscular strength is needed for activities that require a significant or maximal force.

For example, a weightlifter needs good muscular strength to lift heavy weights.

## Strength vs. endurance

Don't get muscular strength confused with MUSCULAR ENDURANCE or POWER – they are all different.

- Muscular strength is about exerting a maximum force and by its very definition could not be done repeatedly, so it is different from muscular endurance.
- Power is about being able to use muscular strength at speed.

## Body composition in sport

BODY COMPOSITION is one of the six components of physical fitness. Athletic success is a combination of body composition and athletic ability.

Body composition will impact on sports performers. Sprinters benefit from having a low ratio of body fat to muscles as a leaner body performs better amd faster, while sumo wrestlers will normally have a higher body fat to muscle ratio as body mass is important to their success.

## Worked example

Look at the images on the right.

Match the images with the appropriate description.
**(2 marks)**

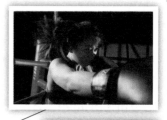

An athlete using muscular power. Muscular power is the ability to use muscular strength at speed.

An athlete using muscular strength. Muscular strength is the maximum force that a muscle is able to exert. It makes no reference to the speed of this exertion.

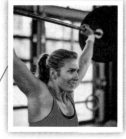

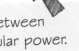

Think about the difference between muscular strength and muscular power.

## Now try this

Complete the table below by giving an example of how muscular strength would be used by each performer.
**(3 marks)**

| Performer | How is muscular strength used? |
|---|---|
| Sprinter | |
| Rugby player | |
| Gymnast | |

# Agility

There are five components of skill-related fitness. Agility is one of these. Agility is the ability of a sports performer to quickly and precisely move or change direction without losing balance or time.

## Agility in action

Sports performers are often required to dodge and move quickly past the opposition to create space and score goals.

This is most common in team sports where there are lots of players in the same space at the same time.

If performers do not have good agility then it is easier for the defence to mark them closely and make tackles, intercept passes and keep them out of the game.

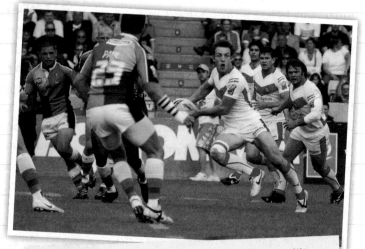

Rugby players need to have good agility in order to change direction quickly and avoid tackles from opposing players.

## When is agility not important?

100 m sprinters do not have to change direction or worry about other players.

## Improving agility

Sports performers can improve their agility by taking part in SPEED, AGILITY, QUICKNESS (SAQ) TRAINING. This involves lots of quick, explosive movements.

---

## Worked example

Describe **one** example that shows why agility may be needed in a sport of your choice.
**(2 marks)**

The question asks for an example. It is a good idea to choose a sport where there are obvious examples so that you can describe one well.

In netball, agility is required by the wing attack in order to dodge away from the wing defence and into space on a centre pass. If the player does not have good agility the defender will be able to keep up with them and is more likely to intercept a pass.

During the online test, you can use the 'review' button to go back and check your answers.

---

## Now try this

When explaining why agility is important, try to give specific examples of when it may be used in a game situation.

Explain why agility is important for a basketball player.
**(2 marks)**

# Balance

Balance is one of the five components of skill-related fitness and can be defined as the ability of a performer to maintain their centre of mass over a base of support. Balance is used in all activities but there are some in which balance is especially important. There are two types of balance.

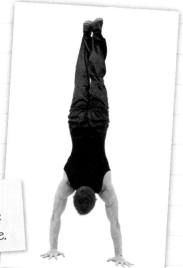

**① Static balance**

STATIC BALANCE is maintaining balance in a STATIONARY position. A gymnast uses static balance during a handstand to hold their position still.

A handstand requires the use of static balance.

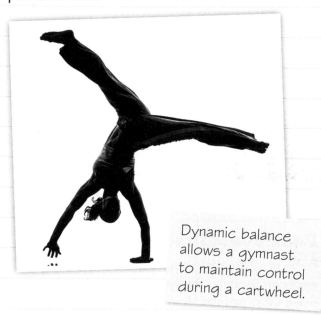

**② Dynamic balance**

DYNAMIC BALANCE is all about a performer's ability to maintain balance while in MOTION; for example, a gymnast's ability to perform a controlled cartwheel or an athlete's ability to run without falling over.

Dynamic balance allows a gymnast to maintain control during a cartwheel.

## Worked example

Which of the following is an example of static balance?    **(1 mark)**

A ☐ A footballer dribbling a ball

B ☑ A headstand

C ☐ A backflip

D ☐ A sprinter competing in the 100 m

In some activities it might not be obvious why balance is important. Think about the activity from start to finish. Is there a time when balance is most important?

## Now try this

Look at the image, which shows an athlete in the discus throw event.

Give **one** example of why balance is important for this athlete.    **(1 mark)**

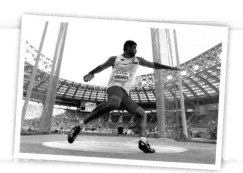

7

# Coordination

Coordination is one of the five components of skill-related fitness and is the ability to use parts of the body together to move smoothly and accurately. Good coordination ensures that tasks are performed efficiently and accurately. There are three types of coordination.

## 1 Hand-eye coordination

Good HAND–EYE COORDINATION is needed in lots of sports. For example, baseball players need to ensure that the bat and ball make contact.

## 2 Foot-eye coordination

Good FOOT–EYE COORDINATION is needed in football to allow the players to watch the ball move towards and away from their feet and keep it under control.

## 3 Hand-to-hand coordination

Good HAND–TO–HAND COORDINATION is needed by a basketball player to switch hands when dribbling the ball.

### Poor coordination

Poor coordination reduces accuracy and can lead to mistakes that can cost vital points. It can also lead to injury during training.

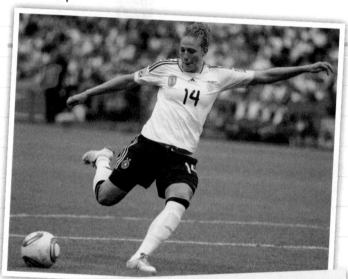

Football players need excellent foot–eye coordination to keep the ball under control.

If a question asks you to 'explain', make sure you give specific examples to support the statement. Make it clear which body parts are working together.

## Worked example

Using a specific sports example, explain how poor coordination may increase the risk of injury. **(2 marks)**

If a gymnast on the beam does not have good coordination they are more likely to misjudge where the beam is and get their foot/hand placement wrong. This increases the chance that they will fall off the beam and injure themselves.

## Now try this

Look at the netball player in the image below.

Give **one** example of when a netball player would use hand-eye coordination in their sport. **(1 mark)**

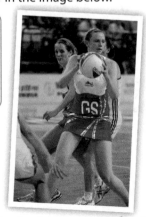

# Power

Power is one of the five components of skill-related fitness. Power is the ability to use strength at speed.

In order to have power you must have both STRENGTH and SPEED.

## Calculating power

Power can be calculated as follows:

POWER = STRENGTH × SPEED

Power is expressed as the work done in the time taken. So the faster or stronger a movement is, the more powerful it will be.

## Power in sport

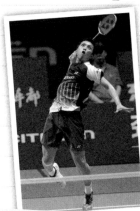

Badminton players use power in a successful smash shot.

Power is important in lots of different activities. Think of activities that have lots of explosive movements in them.

A good example is the smash in badminton. If the player did not have power, the shot would be slower and much easier for the opposition to return. Other examples are a sprinter leaving the starting blocks and a basketball player in a jump shot.

## Physical or skill-related

To be powerful you need to have strength and speed, but also good balance and coordination to direct and control this power.

Make sure you understand how all of the components of fitness are related when you are revising this section.

| Physical fitness | Skill-related fitness |
|---|---|
| Aerobic endurance (page 1) | Agility (page 6) |
| Muscular endurance (page 2) | Balance (page 7) |
| Flexibility (page 3) | Coordination (page 8) |
| Speed (page 4) | Power (this page) |
| Muscular strength (page 5) | Reaction time (page 10) |
| Body composition (page 5) | |

To show your understanding of all the components of fitness, make sure that you can apply the theory to specific physical activities or sports as in the examples given throughout these pages.

## Worked example

Give **three** examples of a specific moment in which an athlete would need power in their sport. Use a different sport for each example. **(3 marks)**

Make sure you give three different examples.

```
1. A sprinter leaving the starting
   blocks
2. A high jumper at take-off
3. A shot putter releasing the shot
```

## Now try this

Lucy is a tennis player. She has been told that she needs to improve her power.

Using an example, explain why power is important to a tennis player. **(2 marks)**

# Reaction time

Reaction time is one of the five components of skill-related fitness and refers to how quickly a sports performer can react or adapt.

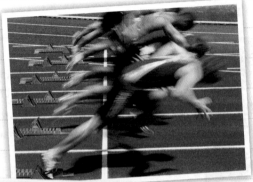

Sprinters need to react quickly to the starting gun to get a good race start.

## What is reaction time?

Reaction time is the time taken for a sports performer to respond to a stimulus and the initiation of this response; for example, the time taken for a 100 m sprinter to hear the starter's gun and then leave their blocks. The shorter this period of time, the faster their reaction time.

Fast reaction time is needed in activities where quick decisions and responses need to be made.

| Who needs it? | When would they use it? |
|---|---|
| Swimmer | To respond quickly to the gun at the start of a race |
| Tennis player | When they realise they are going the wrong way to return a shot and need to change direction |
| Hockey goalkeeper | To block shots accurately |

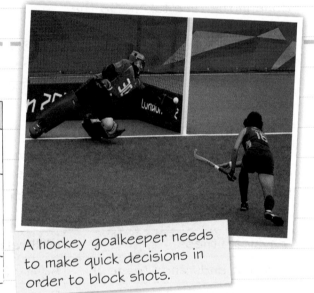

A hockey goalkeeper needs to make quick decisions in order to block shots.

## Worked example

For each performer, give **one** example of how they benefit from a fast reaction time. **(2 marks)**

| Performer | Why is having a fast reaction time important? |
|---|---|
| Badminton player | To decide quickly on the type of return they will play and to initiate the required movement |
| Netball player | Has three seconds to decide how to respond to any pass they receive |

## Now try this

Give **two** examples that demonstrate the importance of quick reaction times in cricket. **(2 marks)**

Think about **two** different playing positions and about when a player in each position might need to respond quickly.

# The importance of fitness components for success in sport

The fitness components covered on the previous pages are important for allowing performers to meet the physical and skill-related demands of particular sports.

It is important to consider the aspects of fitness that are required by different sports performers. This allows you to use appropriate fitness training methods and tests that are specific to the training needs of the individual performer.

## What makes a performer successful?

Look at the table below. It shows why certain performers require certain aspects of fitness in order to be successful.

| Sports performer | Aspects of fitness | Why do they need it? |
|---|---|---|
| 100 m sprinter | Speed, reaction time and power | ✓ Speed: to cover the distance as quickly as possible. <br> ✓ Reaction time: to respond quickly to the starter's pistol. <br> ✓ Power: to move powerfully out of the blocks to get a good start. |
| Football striker | Speed and agility | ✓ Speed: to move quickly into position to receive the ball. They also need good speed endurance to be able to continue to move at speed throughout the game. <br> ✓ Agility: to avoid defenders when in possession of the ball. |
| Football goalkeeper | Reaction time and flexibility | ✓ Reaction time: to be able to get into position quickly to block shots made on the goal. <br> ✓ Flexibility: to manipulate (by extending and bending) their bodies into positions to block shots made on the goal from all directions. |

Don't forget that in some sports the different positions will have different requirements for successful participation!

## Worked example

Which of the following aspects of fitness is **least** important to a boxer?

A ☐ Power

B ☐ Muscular endurance in the arms

C ☐ Balance

D ☑ Flexibility

## Now try this

Identify **one** example when coordination is important to a squash player.

**(1 mark)**

11

# Exercise intensity: heart rate

Exercise intensity refers to how hard you are working during a training session. Measuring heart rate is one way of measuring exercise intensity.

## Target heart rate

TARGET HEART RATE is the recommended maximum heart rate appropriate for a training zone or physical activity and is the most common method used for measuring exercise intensity. You need a different target heart rate depending on what you are trying to achieve. A target heart rate is the optimal heart rate you need to achieve in order to get specific training adaptations.

Heart rate can be measured manually by counting the pulse or by using a heart rate monitor.

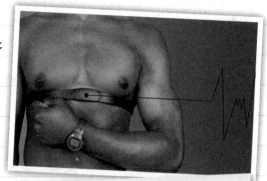
Using a heart rate monitor to measure exercise intensity.

## Why is intensity important?

It is important to get the intensity of your training correct. Training at the wrong intensity may not help to improve the element of fitness you are trying to develop. Training at too high an intensity can result in injury.

## Key terms

You need to understand the following terms in relation to exercise intensity:

HEART RATE (HR): the number of times your heart beats per minute. It is measured in beats per minute (bpm).

RESTING HEART RATE: your heart rate at rest.

MAXIMUM HEART RATE (HRmax): the maximum recommended safe heart rate for an individual during exercise.

## Calculating maximum heart rate

You need to be able to calculate your maximum heart rate as this will help you to work out your training zones and thresholds (see page 14).

In order to estimate your maximum heart rate, you need to use the following formula:

$$\text{MAXIMUM HEART RATE} = 220 - \text{AGE}$$

This means that if Bobby is 18 his maximum heart rate would be 202 bpm:

$$220 - 18 = 202$$

## Worked example

The table below shows the ages for three individuals.

Calculate their HRmax using this information. **(3 marks)**

| Athlete | Age | HRmax |
|---------|-----|-------|
| Rob | 19 | 220 - 19 = 201 |
| Nadeem | 30 | 220 - 30 = 190 |
| Aoife | 54 | 220 - 54 = 166 |

## Now try this

Jane is a 33-year-old female athlete.

What is Jane's maximum heart rate (HRmax) in beats per minute (bpm)? **(2 marks)**

Remember to show your workings when doing calculations. You'll be given a box to show your workings in the online test.

# Exercise intensity: the Borg (RPE) scale

Exercise intensity refers to how hard you are working in a training session. You need to be able to explain what the 'rating of perceived exertion' (RPE) scale measures, and how it can be used to measure exercise intensity and calculate heart rate.

## The Borg Rating of Perceived Exertion (RPE) scale

The Borg (RPE) scale measures a performer's rate of perceived exertion – that is, how hard they think they are working.

It is a scale from 6 to 20, where 6 is no exertion at all and 20 is maximum exertion.

Alongside other physiological data it can be used to estimate HEART RATE (HR) and therefore monitor if a person is in the correct training zone, i.e. if they are working at the appropriate intensity.

It is generally agreed that ratings of perceived exertion between 12 and 14 on the scale suggest that physical activity is being performed at a moderate level of intensity. That would mean that AEROBIC ENDURANCE was being improved.

| Rating of perceived exertion | Intensity |
|---|---|
| 6 | No exertion |
| 7 | |
| 8 | |
| 9 | |
| 10 | |
| 11 | Light |
| 12 | |
| 13 | Somewhat hard |
| 14 | |
| 15 | Hard (heavy) |
| 16 | |
| 17 | Very hard |
| 18 | |
| 19 | |
| 20 | Maximal exertion |

The Borg (1970) 6–20 RPE scale.

## Using the Borg (RPE) scale to predict heart rate

Instead of using a heart rate monitor, you can use the RPE scale to predict the exercise HR of an individual using the formula:

RPE × 10 = HEART RATE (bpm)

If an athlete rates themselves at 14 on the RPE scale this would suggest a heart rate of approximately 140 bpm. This can help you to calculate training zones.

## Example: Luca

Luca has been playing football for an hour. He rates his exercise intensity as 'hard' as he has been running a lot. He thinks he is at 15 on the Borg (RPE) scale.

This means that his exercise HR is:

15 × 10 = 150 bpm.

## Worked example

An individual reports an RPE of 13.

What is their approximate heart rate at this point?    **(1 mark)**

A ☐ 120     B ☑ 130
C ☐ 140     D ☐ 145

Think about the situations you might be in when using the RPE scale.

## Now try this

State **one** benefit of using the Borg (RPE) scale to assess perceived exertion and intensity.    **(1 mark)**

# Exercise intensity: training zones

You will need to be able to explain and calculate training zones.

## Training within your target zones

To maximise the training adaptations taking place during exercise you should train within your TARGET HEART RATE zone.

The target zone you train within depends on the type of benefits you are hoping to achieve.

If you are trying to improve your aerobic endurance then you need to train within your aerobic training zone, which is 60–85 per cent of your MAXIMUM HEART RATE (HRmax).

If you are training for more explosive, high intensity activities you would need to be working within the ANAEROBIC or HIGH INTENSITY training zone. The chart opposite shows the various training zones.

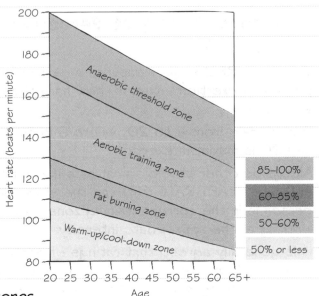

## Calculating your target zones

Your target zones will depend on your age. You need to work out your maximum heart rate and then calculate 60–85 per cent of this total.

Always start with the figure 220.

220 – your age (or the age of the person who is doing the training) = HRmax

↓

Calculate 60 per cent and 85 per cent of this total to give two figures.

↓

These two figures are the two limits of your aerobic training zone. Your heart rate needs to stay within these limits to improve aerobic endurance.

Lucy is 15 years old.
The calculation for her target zone is:

220 − 15 = 205 (HRmax)

↓

60 × 205 ÷ 100 = 123 (60%)
85 × 205 ÷ 100 = 174 (85%)

↓

Therefore Lucy's aerobic training zone is between 123 and 174 bpm.

Keep practising calculations like these and **always** check your workings!

Nigel is 45 years old.

What is the **upper** limit of his aerobic training zone? **(2 marks)**

Please show your calculations.

```
The upper limit of Nigel's aerobic training zone
would be 149 bpm. This is because:
220 − 45 = 175 bpm (HRmax)
85 × 175 ÷ 100 = 149 bpm
```

**Now try this**

What would be the recommended training zone for cardiovascular health and fitness of a 16 year old?

**(2 marks)**

# Basic principles of training

Once you have identified the aspect(s) of fitness that you want to improve, you need to start planning appropriate training. This involves using the FITT principle which helps you plan appropriate training to improve your fitness.

## The FITT principle

FREQUENCY – how often you train

INTENSITY – how hard you train

TIME – how long you train

TYPE – how specific your training should be.

## Planning your training

The FITT principle helps to ensure that you are working at a level that is challenging enough to push the body to make fitness improvements. If you are not working hard enough, your body will not adapt and your fitness will not improve. It is important not to increase any of the elements too quickly as this can lead to burnout and increases the risk of injury.

 ## FITT: Frequency

The number of training sessions completed over a period of time, usually per week. It should be gradually increased over time.

| 1 session | 2 sessions | 3 sessions |
|---|---|---|
| Week 1 | Week 2 | Week 3 |

 ## FITT: Intensity

This is about how hard you train. It should be gradually increased over time.

| 1 set of 5 reps (5 kg) | 2 sets of 5 reps (5 kg) | 2 sets of 5 reps (10 kg) |
|---|---|---|
| Session 1 | Session 3 | Session 5 |

 ## FITT: Time

This is about how long you train for. It should be gradually increased over time.

| 20 mins | 25 mins | 30 mins |
|---|---|---|
| Session 1 | Session 3 | Session 5 |

 ## FITT: Type

This is related to the principle of specificity (see page 16).
If a training method is selected to improve a specific component of fitness there is more likely to be a positive improvement in performance.

## Worked example

Elle has started circuit training to help improve her general fitness. After a month, she thinks that her circuit training sessions could last longer, starting at 20 minutes and then moving to 30 minutes, so that she better benefits from the training.

> Which part of the FITT principle is being referred to in this statement? **(1 mark)**

> The 'time' principle as Elle is increasing the length of time she trains each week.

## Now try this

Aylin is planning a training programme to develop her aerobic endurance for swimming.

> Describe how Aylin should apply **one** of the FITT principles to this training programme. **(2 marks)**

# Additional principles of training 1

You need to be able to define the principles of training and explain how they would be applied in a practical context.

SPECIFICITY means that training should be specific to the individual's sport, activity or fitness-related goals.

The principle of specificity is about matching training to the particular requirements of your activity, making sure that training is relevant to your sport or the fitness goals you are trying to achieve. This is so that you train the appropriate muscles in the right way, rather than working on other aspects of fitness that may not help to improve your performance.

Don't get specificity confused with individual needs – specificity is about the requirements of the activity and not the person.

Specific training for a sprint cyclist could be using an exercise bike in a gym – a better match than a treadmill or a rowing machine.

## Applying the specificity principle to training

You need to think about the fitness requirements of your sport to decide on the most appropriate specific training. For example:

- it would be appropriate for a 100 m sprinter to do speed training on a track or to work on sprint starts because these activities are directly relevant to a sprinting event
- it wouldn't be appropriate for a discus thrower to do speed training on a track as this activity is not relevant to their sport
- specific training for a swimmer would be more likely to be based in a swimming pool, to work muscles in the same way as in swimming events
- specific training for a football player could involve fartlek training in a local park.

### Worked example

Josh is a middle-distance runner. His coach has suggested that he should do some training at his local swimming pool.

Using the principle of specificity, explain if this is appropriate training. **(2 marks)**

The training is not appropriate because Josh is a runner, therefore if he swims he will be training the wrong muscles and will not be improving his fitness for running so will not improve his performance.

### Now try this

Look at the images on the right, which show three different pieces of fitness equipment.

For each piece of equipment, state **one** sporting activity for which it would be an appropriate method of training.
**(3 marks)**

Think about what each piece of equipment specifically exercises and then think about who that would be useful to.

| Fitness equipment | Appropriate sporting activity |
|---|---|
| 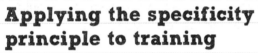 Rowing machine | |
| Exercise bike | |
| Treadmill | |

# Additional principles of training 2

Training needs to be demanding enough to cause the body to adapt. In order to make fitness gains, training must get more demanding over time – this is called PROGRESSIVE OVERLOAD.

It is important that overload is applied gradually to reduce the risk of injury.

Progressive overload can be applied by using the FITT principles and gradually increasing the:

- FREQUENCY of training
- INTENSITY of training
- length (TIME) of training.

Someone training for a half marathon could apply this principle to their training by gradually:

- ✓ running further, or
- ✓ running for longer, or
- ✓ running at a slightly faster pace, or
- ✓ running more often.

It is important not to use all these methods at once, as the increase in workload could lead to overtraining.

It is important to overload but not to overtrain. Overtraining can result in injury or illness.

## Increasing intensity

In a fitness training programme, progressive overload can be applied by increasing the intensity of training. It might look like this:

     Week 1 = do 10 pull-ups

     Week 2 = do 15 pull-ups

     Week 3 = do 20 pull-ups

## The plateau

If an athlete trains regularly but at the same intensity for a prolonged period of time, their body will become used to the load being placed on it. This is known as the TRAINING PLATEAU.

## Worked example

What is the difference between overload and overtraining?    **(2 marks)**

Insert the correct term next to each definition.

| Overload | is the process of making your body work harder than it is used to in order to improve specific aspects of fitness.

| Overtraining | is pushing yourself beyond your capabilities and is more likely to result in an injury.

 Make sure you learn the difference between these terms.

## Now try this

 Think about overload over time – how would you apply the FITT principle to this question?

Using a sporting example, explain the principle of progressive overload.    **(2 marks)**

Always make sure you use relevant examples.

# Additional principles of training 3

All fitness training programmes should be designed to meet the training needs and goals of the INDIVIDUAL. Programmes should be designed specifically for the individual, taking into account differences.

## Individual differences/needs

If one person wants to improve their speed and agility while another wants to improve their aerobic endurance, their training needs would be very different.

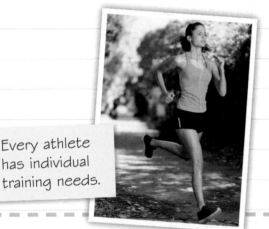

Every athlete has individual training needs.

Health status    Fitness goals

Access to equipment    **Individual differences /needs**    Prior fitness levels

Availability of time    Sport/activity

Injury    Personal heart rate zone

---

This is all about the individual needs of the performer – you must ensure that the training programme chosen will help them to meet their individual fitness goals.

### Worked example

Anna is a netball player and wants to develop explosive power in her quadriceps to help increase her jumping height.

Why would a speed training programme **not** be appropriate?    **(2 marks)**

```
Training needs to be tailored to meet
the individual needs of the performer.
Speed training, although appropriate
to netball, would not help Anna meet
her specific training goal as well as a
training programme such as plyometric
training that included jumps.
```

## Lifestyle factors

Certain lifestyle factors such as working hours, cost and access to specialised facilities may impact on an individual's training needs.

If someone is working during the day they would need to have access to training early in the morning or in the evening. This would be an individual need.

### Individual vs. specific

INDIVIDUAL training needs are not the same as SPECIFIC training needs. Individual training needs are about the person; specific training needs are about the activity or sport.

---

### Now try this

(a) State **two** lifestyle factors that may impact on a person's access to exercise.    **(2 marks)**

Think about what would affect your own exercise routine.

(b) Outline the potential impact of these factors on an individual's training needs.    **(2 marks)**

# Addditional principles of training 4

Your body will respond to training by ADAPTING and improving its ability to cope with increased training loads, but this process can also be REVERSED if training stops.

## Adaptation

Adaptation happens during the recovery period following a training session. It is the way your body increases its ability to cope with training loads.

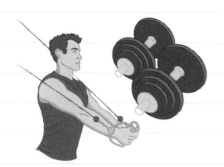

Weight training causes the body to adapt muscle size and increase strength.

## Reversibility

Just as fitness can be improved with regular training, it can also be lost if training is stopped, for example as a result of injury or if the INTENSITY of the training is not sufficient to cause adaptation. Reversibility is also known as de-training.

## Muscular adaptations

MUSCULAR HYPERTROPHY is an example of an adaptation related to weight training. Over time, training results in an increase in the number and size of muscular cells called myofibrils. This increases the size of the muscle and results in an increase in strength.

A loss in muscular size and strength is called MUSCULAR ATROPHY.

## Rest and recovery

Rest is the period of time provided for recovery to take place. It is important to allow enough time to recover as this is when training adaptations occur. Recovery also allows damage to be repaired and energy stores to be replenished.

By not allowing for rest and recovery you run the risk of overtraining. This can cause a drop in performance due to insufficient time for rest and recovery and increases the risk of injury.

## Worked example

Which of these is **not** a reason for rest and recovery in training?          **(1 mark)**

A ☐ Positive training adaptations

B ☑ Reduce blood pressure

C ☐ Repair damage

D ☐ Replenish energy

## Now try this

Explain the difference between adaptation and reversibility.          **(2 marks)**

For 'explain' questions you should write a few sentences. Identify the main difference and then expand your answer.

# Additional principles of training 5

It is important to add VARIATION to training routines to avoid boredom and maintain enjoyment.

## Varying training routines

Minor changes in routine can produce large fitness gains. This change is known as variation.

Some basic things that could be done to ensure variation include changing the:

- type of equipment
- training environment
- order of training
- type of exercise
- nature of your training.

## Why is variation important?

Variation is important because it helps to:

✓ keep you interested and maintain the motivation and enjoyment associated with training. If you are doing the same training all the time you are likely to become bored and so more likely to give up.

✓ provide new challenges for your body and reduces the risk of injuries caused by the repetition of the same actions and training methods.

## Variation in practice

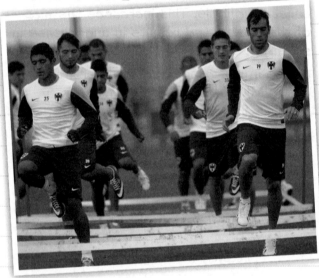

You still need to consider the specificity principle (see page 16) so that any variation is beneficial to the individual and their training goals.

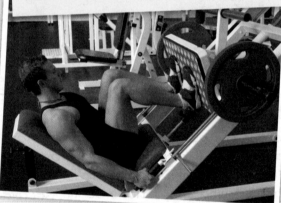

An example of variation in practice is a footballer who uses both bounding ladder drills and weight training to help build both leg power and strength. This will allow for recovery and adaptation to take place whilst maintaining enjoyment. This way he is more likely to persist with his training.

Think about all the different training programmes before you answer this question.

Neelesh is training on his own to improve his aerobic endurance.

> Give **two** examples of how variation can be applied to reduce boredom in his training. **(2 marks)**

> Neelesh could change his training location for one session a week. Instead of running on the road he could run on a treadmill in the gym. He could also try running as part of a group rather than on his own.

> Give **two** reasons why variation in training is important. **(2 marks)**

Think about how you would feel if you did the same training all the time.

# Circuit training

A sports performer's training routine can include lots of different training methods. Circuit training involves a series of different activities that can be either sport-specific or tailored to improve certain aspects of fitness. Circuit training can be adapted to suit the fitness needs of the individual. It can also be used to improve general fitness.

## Features of circuit training

Multiple stations

Can be used to develop all aspects of fitness – depending on the stations chosen

Can be fitness-based or sport specific

Can be either aerobic or anaerobic depending on intensity

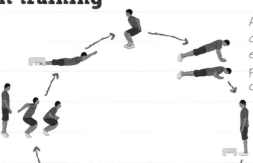

A warm-up should always be completed. Some cardiovascular exercises, such as light jogging, plus stretching, should be carried out before circuit training.

Activities are done for 30–60 seconds

30–60 seconds is allowed for moving between stations

## Increasing intensity

Intensity can be increased by:
- increasing the time at each station
- increasing the number of circuits completed
- adding extra stations.

Advantage: can be adapted to suit any fitness level or any type of sport.

Disadvantage: often requires lots of space and specialised equipment.

## Variation

The exercises at circuit stations should be varied so that muscles have time to recover. To reduce the risk of injury you should never exercise the same body part or muscles consecutively.

## Now try this

Emma is 15 years old. She has designed a circuit to help improve her performance in netball. The images below show each of the four stations:

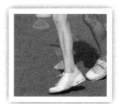

Station 1 – running in and out of cones

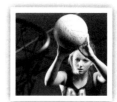

Station 2 – shots into a netball ring

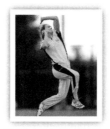

Station 3 – bowling at a target

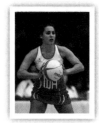

Station 4 – chest passes at a wall

## Worked example

Ghalib wants to improve his upper-body muscular endurance.

Give **three** examples of stations that would be appropriate for him to include in a circuit.
**(3 marks)**

Sit-ups, tricep dips, back raises.

Remember the **principle of specificity** when answering this question. Which stations will help Emma improve her performance at netball?

Circle the station that isn't appropriate for her circuit. **(1 mark)**

# Continuous training

A sports performer's training routine can include lots of different training methods. Continuous training is a steady pace, moderate-intensity training method used for developing aerobic endurance.

## Characteristics of continuous training

It involves working at a steady pace for at least 30 minutes with no breaks.

Running at a steady pace for 30 minutes around a running track without stopping is an example of continuous training.

Continuous training must be performed in the correct training zone. This is 60–85 per cent of your maximum heart rate. (Remind yourself how to calculate training zones by looking at page 14.)

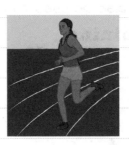

Continuous training activities include long distance:
- running
- cycling
- swimming.

This training is great for triathletes.

### Uses of continuous training

Continuous training can be:
- good sport-specific training for marathon runners and long-distance swimmers
- useful for team sport players (e.g. netball/hockey) who might use continuous training as a part of their training routine
- a useful training method for people who have a lower level of fitness
- used to reduce the risk of high blood pressure and coronary heart disease.

### Applying the FITT principle
- Run more often (frequency)
- Run for longer (time)
- Run at a faster pace (intensity).

## Benefits and disadvantages of continuous training

| Benefits | Disadvantages |
|---|---|
| ✓ Easy to organise and do | ✗ Training for long distances can be boring |
| ✓ Requires little equipment | ✗ Only develops aerobic endurance, not anaerobic |
| ✓ Can be done anywhere | ✗ Higher risk of injury if running on a hard surface |
| ✓ Can be made sport-specific | ✗ Not ideal for a team sport player (e.g. handball/ rugby) as it does not improve speed |
| ✓ Improves aerobic endurance | |
| ✓ Improves muscular endurance | |
| ✓ Good for beginners | |

Continuous training can result in overuse injuries, such as shin splints, so it is important to add variation to your training. This variation also helps to reduce boredom.

## Worked example

Which of these athletes is most likely to use continuous training as their main training method?   **(1 mark)**

A ☐ Dancer    B ✓ Long-distance cyclist

C ☐ Gymnast   D ☐ Rugby player

## Now try this

Colin is 34 years old.

Calculate Colin's target heart rate zone for a continuous training regime.   **(4 marks)**

Remind yourself how to calculate **target heart rate** zones by revising page 14.

# Fartlek training

A sports performer's training routine can include lots of different training methods. Fartlek training is a form of continuous training where intensity is changed by running at different speeds or over different terrains.

## How fartlek training works

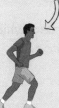 Performer can work maximally

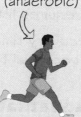 Sprinting (anaerobic)

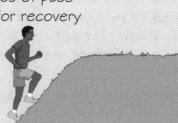 Changes of pace allow for recovery

Changes of pace allow for recovery.

It improves aerobic and muscular endurance and reduces the chance of coronary heart disease.

It is continuous, but the changes in intensity can help to improve both aerobic and anaerobic performance.

## Increasing intensity

There are no rest periods in fartlek training.

You can further increase the intensity of fartlek training by using weighted vests and running harnesses.

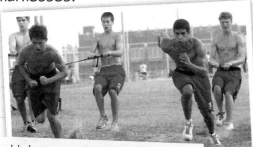

Using a running harness increases training intensity.

## Adapting fartlek training

Fartlek training can be adapted easily to suit the individual's level of personal fitness and training method. It can be performed on a bike if you are a cyclist or in the pool if you are a swimmer.

It is a good training method for sports team players who need to be able to cope with changes of pace in competition as it helps to improve both aerobic and anaerobic fitness.

## Be prepared

- Good running shoes are important if you are running on varied terrains.
- A good warm-up and cool-down are important.

Make sure you think about what can be changed specifically in fartlek training.

## Worked example

A cross-country runner decides to include fartlek training in their training programme.

Explain how they might adapt fartlek training to suit their activity. **(2 marks)**

A cross-country runner would focus on changing terrains and inclines to match the conditions they would find in competition.

## Now try this

You take part in a team sport (e.g. football).

Explain why you should focus on changing speeds rather than terrains in a fartlek session. **(2 marks)**

Think about what a football pitch looks like. What type of terrain is it?

# Interval training

A sports performer's training routine can include lots of different training methods. Interval training is where periods of exercising are followed by a rest or recovery period.

## Characteristics

Interval training involves periods of high intensity exercise, training for 30 seconds to 5 minutes, followed by periods of rest or lower intensity work. These rest periods allow for recovery and can be complete rest, walking or light jogging.

Interval training is most commonly associated with explosive power activities such as sprinting and weight lifting; however, it can be adapted to develop other aspects of fitness.

> Strength could be improved if breaks are programmed into a weight training session, for example:
> • 10 reps arms, rest arms
> • 10 reps legs, rest legs
> • 10 reps arms, rest arms.

## Advantages

✓ It can be used to develop a number of fitness components, such as aerobic endurance.

✓ It requires little equipment.

✓ Recovery time gets shorter, which is beneficial to performance.

## Disadvantages

✗ You need to make sure that you keep working hard when you start to fatigue, which isn't easy.

✗ There is also a real risk of overtraining that can cause injuries. Always add variation to this training to help avoid this.

## Intervals for aerobic endurance

If you want to improve aerobic endurance, make the periods of work longer but perform them at a moderate intensity. Typical work intervals will be around 60% maximumn oxygen uptake (VO$_2$ max).

> To increase intensity you would decrease the number of rest periods but continue to work at an intensity within the aerobic training zone. Remember that this is the intensity part of the FITT principle.

## Intervals for speed

If you want to improve your speed or power, use shorter work intervals and perform close to your maximum intensity.

> To increase intensity you would reduce the length or number of rest periods and increase the intensity of the work periods.

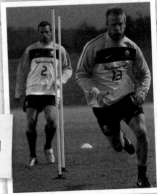

Sprint drills are a form of interval training.

## Worked example

Interval training is a method of training that can be used by a variety of performers.

> Which **two** of the following are characteristics of interval training? **(2 marks)**
>
> A ☑ Periods of work followed by periods of rest
> B ☑ Running at different intensities
> C ☐ Running over different terrains
> D ☐ Working for 30 minutes with no breaks
> E ☐ Accelerating over a 20 minute run

If you want to come back to a question in the online test, click the 'flag' button.

## Now try this

Explain how you could tell by looking at a performer's interval training session plan if they were an endurance or power athlete. **(2 marks)**

# Plyometric training

A sports performer's training routine can include lots of different training methods. Plyometric training develops sport-specific explosive power and strength.

## How plyometric training is used

Plyometric training can be used to develop power and speed as well as sport-specific skills. It involves lots of explosive movements and works by making muscles exert their maximal force in a short time period.

Plyometric training involves exercises that make the muscles contract and relax rapidly.

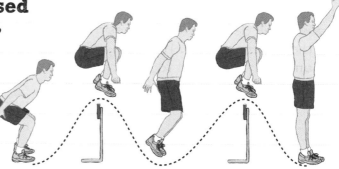

Hurdling is a type of plyometric exercise.

## Types of plyometric exercises

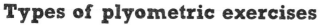

There are a number of exercises you can do as part of your training: bounding, lunges, inclined press-ups, hurdle jumping, press-ups with claps.

An intense warm-up is vital to prevent injury and to warm muscles up thoroughly.

Intensity can be increased by increasing the number of repetitions of an exercise, this should be done carefully as this training is intense and so can result in injury.

Sports performers that benefit from plyometric training are:

* sprinters – they need explosive power at take-off when they hear the starting gun
* hurdlers – they need to jump over hurdles while maintaining speed
* volleyball players – they need to jump high and contest the ball.

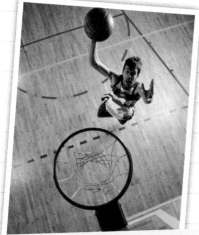

Plyometric training is useful for basketball players.

## How it works

It is important to learn and practise the techniques for plyometric training as it can be physically stressful and cause muscle soreness. Exercises need to be performed on a suitable surface that will absorb some of the force being produced. Plyometric exercises need maximal force as the muscle lengthens (eccentric action) before an immediate maximal force as the muscle shortens (concentric action).

Advantage: can be adapted to suit a variety of sports.

Disadvantages: not suitable for young athletes and need to be careful with techniques to avoid injury.

## Worked example

State **one** way plyometric training could be incorporated into the training routine of a rugby player? **(1 mark)**

Plyometric training can be organised as part of a circuit training session with stations such as box jumps and inclined press-ups.

## Now try this

Explain how plyometric training helps to prepare an athlete for a sport-specific performance of your choice. **(2 marks)**

# Speed training methods

A sports performer's training routine can include lots of different training methods. Speed training takes different forms and can be made sport-specific.

The type of speed training an athlete chooses will depend on their sport and their fitness goals. For example, if a long jumper wanted to improve their speed on their run-up they would choose acceleration sprint training.

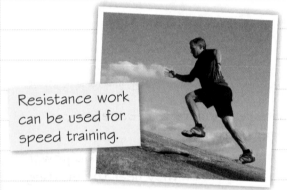

Resistance work can be used for speed training.

## ① Acceleration sprints

- Pace is increased gradually from standing or rolling to jogging, then striding, and then to a maximum sprint.
- Different drills, such as resistance work and hill runs, can be used.
- Rest intervals of jogging or walking are used between each repetition.
- They are a good form of anaerobic training.

## ③ Interval training

- A work period is followed by a rest or recovery period.
- To develop speed, work intervals will be short and performed at a high intensity.
- Speed is developed by increasing work intensity and the number of rest periods.
- Intervals vary depending on the individual athlete's goals. For example:
  - 100 m sprinter: 10 × 30 m @ race pace
  - 800 m runner: 5 × 200 m @ goal race pace

## ② Hollow sprints

- A series of sprints is followed by 'hollow' periods of jogging or walking.
- They are useful for football players who need constant changes of speed during a game.

---

### Applying the FITT principle

Overload can be achieved by reducing the length of the rest period and increasing the length or intensity of the work periods. Intensity can be increased by running up hills or along more challenging terrain.

Advantages: need little specialist equipment and can be adapted to suit an individual's training needs.

Disadvantages: it can become tedious and so should be used with other training methods.

---

### Worked example

Which type of speed training method would be most appropriate for a hockey player?
**(1 mark)**

A ☐ Interval training

B ☐ Resistance training

C ☑ Hollow sprints

D ☐ Acceleration sprints

Think about a car accelerating away from stationary – can you use this action to help you answer the question?

### Now try this

Outline **one** difference between acceleration sprints and hollow sprints. **(1 mark)**

# Flexibility training

Flexibility is important for all sports performers. The principle of specifity should be applied to flexibility training – you should stretch the muscle groups that will be used in your sport. There are three types of flexibility training methods.

## ① Static stretching

STATIC STRETCHING helps you to reduce the risk of muscle soreness and injury. There are two types of static flexibility training; active and passive:

1 ACTIVE STRETCHING is performed independently and uses internal force to stretch and lengthen the muscle.

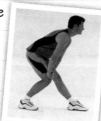
Active stretching.

2 PASSIVE STRETCHING requires the help of another person or object to provide external force, causing the muscle to stretch.

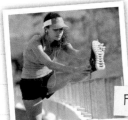
Passive stretching.

## ② Ballistic stretching

BALLISTIC STRETCHING uses the force of limb movement to stretch muscles beyond their normal range of movement.

The movements are fast and jerky and usually involve bouncing through the full range of movement. These types of bouncing movements mean that there is the potential for injury.

Ballistic stretching can incorporate sport-specific movements and can form a useful part of a warm-up.

## ③ Proprioceptive neuromuscular facilitation (PNF)

- PNF is an advanced form of passive stretching, using a partner or object to provide resistance.
- PNF is used to develop flexibility, mobility and strength.
- It is often used in rehabilitation programmes when recovering from injury.
- The stretch is held at its upper limit for 6–10 seconds.

- The stretch is enhanced by ISOMETRICALLY contracting the muscle you are stretching. In the stretch shown in the image above, this would involve pushing the left leg against the object.
- After 10 seconds the muscle is relaxed from the isometric contraction and stretched further with the help of a partner or object.
- The process is then repeated.

### Warm-up

All sports performers should conduct some form of flexibility training as part of their WARM-UP to reduce the risk of injury.

Performers such as gymnasts and hurdlers use flexibility training as part of their warm-up in order to improve performance.

## Worked example

Outline **one** difference between passive stretching and PNF. **(1 mark)**

Passive stretching is normally used as part of a warm-up, whereas PNF is most often used in sports rehabilitation.

## Now try this

What type of flexibility training is this athlete performing? **(1 mark)**

A ☐ PNF
B ☐ Ballistic stretching
C ☐ Active stretching
D ☐ Passive stretching

# Weight training

Weight training is a form of interval training. It involves using reps (the number of times the weight is lifted) and sets of reps (for example, 3 sets of 12 reps).

## Purpose of weight training

- To develop STRENGTH – low reps but high load.
- To develop ENDURANCE – high reps but low load.

## 1 rep max (1RM)

1RM refers to the maximum amount of weight a person can lift in a single repetition of a given exercise.

Intensity can be set using a percentage of this figure.

## Maintaining safety

You should always follow the correct guidelines when using weights. Using the correct weight and technique will help reduce the risk of injury.

## A typical programme

**1** Focus on core exercises (working muscles that help to stabilise the spine and pelvis)

**2** Assistance exercises (working specific muscles for a performer's sport or training programme)

**3** Alternate between upper and lower body exercises and alternate between push and pull exercises.

### Applying the FITT principle

- Increase the resistance.
- Increase the number of reps.
- Increase the number of sets.

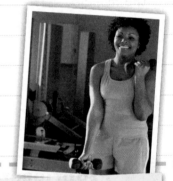

The use of dumb-bells and barbells allow people to perform different dynamic exercises.

| Training for | Percentage of 1RM and number of reps | Used for |
|---|---|---|
| Strength endurance | 50–60% of 1RM and 20 reps | Repetitive movements of a muscle, e.g. cycling |
| Elastic strength | 75% of 1RM and 12 reps | Producing movements in quick succession, e.g. gymnastics |
| Maximum strength | 90% of 1RM and 6 reps | Single movements against a load, e.g. shot put |

Allow time for recovery to reduce risk of injury and allow adaptations to occur. The intensity of training and weight lifted will depend on individual goals.

### Example: Shot-putter

A shot-putter would want to develop their maximum strength as this is crucial to their event. To achieve this they would train using heavy weights for a low number of reps.

Advantages: can be adapted to different performers.

Disadvantges: requires specialised equipment. If used incorrectly can cause injury.

## Worked example

Emil wants to develop his elastic strength. His 1RM is 135 kg.

> What would be an approximate weight for him to lift to improve his elastic strength?
>
> **(2 marks)**

`75% of 135 = 12 reps of 101.25 kg`

## Now try this

> Give **two** reasons why it is important to have a recovery period after weight training.
>
> **(2 marks)**

# Fitness testing: importance to sports performers and coaches

When thinking about why we test fitness, don't forget to think about before, during and after the training programme – you need to be able to monitor whether the training is working.

## Baseline data

Fitness testing provides BASELINE data from which we can monitor and improve performance.

Baseline data are the scores recorded at the start of any training programme.

For example, a gymnast's coach might record baseline data for flexibility, strength and speed. Over time these tests can be repeated, helping to show improvements and areas for further attention.

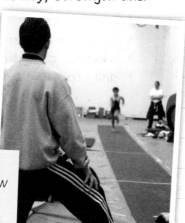

Baseline data for a gymnast might show flexibility, strength and speed.

## Training programmes

Coaches can use baseline data to design training programmes based on a performer's strengths and weaknesses.

If a sprinter has good speed but their reaction time is below average, it gives the coach and athlete an area of training to focus on.

Fitness testing also allows you to see if training programmes are working. By repeating the same tests before and after a training block you can see if programmes have been effective.

### FITT principle

After test results, coaches will use the FITT principle to plan training programmes.

See page 15 to remind yourself of the FITT principle.

## Goal setting

Fitness testing results can provide performers with something to aim for and allow them to set themselves goals. This can be motivating and will encourage them to work hard in training. For example, a netball wing attack may set themselves a target of improving their Illinois agility run test scores by 3 seconds over a 6-week training period (see page 39). By testing at regular intervals they will be able to see their progress towards this goal.

### Learn these!

The following pages of this revision guide cover various fitness tests. Make sure you are able to describe how each test is carried out, what it measures and who might use it.

### Worked example

State **one** reason why it is important to record baseline fitness scores. **(1 mark)**

Baseline scores are important because they provide you with something to compare further test scores against.

### Now try this

What might a coach do if an athlete's post-training programme test results showed no improvement? **(1 mark)**

A ☐ Consider changing the frequency, intensity, time or type of training as it currently might not be appropriate

B ☐ Repeat the same training programme but make the performer take longer rest breaks

C ☐ Repeat the same training programme but make the performer train for longer

D ☐ Consider changing the equipment that the performer has been using

WITHDRAWN from College LRC

THE BOURNEMOUTH & POOLE COLLEGE

29

# Fitness testing: issues, validity and reliability

Various fitness tests are available to test all aspects of physical and skill-related fitness. You need to be aware of the requirements for performing fitness tests and know how to assess the validity and reliability of tests.

## Validity

VALIDITY is how ACCURATE a set of results are. That is, do the results really measure what we want them to?

### Example: Ceri

Ceri weighs herself on a set of scales. When she gets off the scales, she notices that they do not go back to zero. Therefore when she weighs herself again she does not get a true reading of her weight – the result is not valid.

## Reliability

RELIABILITY is the ability to REPEATEDLY carry out the same test and expect comparable results each time.

Things that can influence reliability are:
- length and type of warm-up
- time of day
- amount of sleep the subject has had
- weather conditions
- daily food and drink intake.

## Practicality

PRACTICALITY refers to how suitable the test is for the given situation. Things to consider might be the space required for the test or any specialist equipment that is needed. Some tests may be more practical than others.

Fitness tests should always be valid and reliable.

### Informed consent

This should be gathered from anyone taking part in a fitness test. People being tested must clearly understand the nature of the test and what it will involve. They also have the right to back out at any time. Depending on the age of the person being tested, parental consent may need to be given.

### Calibration

This is the process of checking, and if necessary adjusting, pieces of fitness testing equipment to ensure they are accurate. Equipment should be calibrated regularly to ensure results are valid and accurate.

## Worked example

Think about any fitness tests you have taken and how they were kept valid **and** reliable.

Discuss how it may be possible for a test to be valid but not reliable.  **(2 marks)**

If an athlete uses a hand grip dynamometer to measure strength and they use the same calibrated piece of equipment each time, the results will be valid because the measurements will always be starting from the same base point. But if this athlete completes the test twice, once in the morning and once after a hard day's training, the results would not be reliable as fatigue is likely to impact on the quality of the second result.

## Now try this

You are working as a fitness coach for a football team. Having completed the multistage fitness test six weeks ago, you want to test again to check for improvements.

State **three** things you should consider to ensure the test is reliable. **(3 marks)**

# Fitness tests: skinfold testing (body composition 1)

Skinfold testing is one of three tests used to measure body composition.

## Characteristics of skinfold testing

- Measures: percentage body fat
- Equipment: skinfold callipers and an assistant

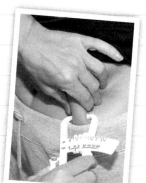

## Method

1. Measurements should be taken on dry skin on the right-hand side of the body.
2. Grasp the skinfold between the thumb and index finger. Mark skinfold sites with a pen.
3. Place the callipers over the fold and release the handles.
4. Read the measurement (in mm) from the dial. Keep hold of the skinfold during the measurement.
5. Repeat measurements at each site three times at 15 second intervals. Take an average.

### Where to measure

To ensure VALIDITY take measurements in exactly the same place each time.

| Males | Females |
|---|---|
| Chest | Tricep |
| Thigh | Suprailiac (hip) |
| Abdomen | Thigh |

## Calculating results using the Jackson-Pollock nomogram

- Add up the sum of your skinfold measurements.
- Plot your age in years and your total sum body fat onto the Jackson-Pollock (J-P) nomogram.
- Join the two lines up using a ruler.
- Read your percentage body fat according to your gender.

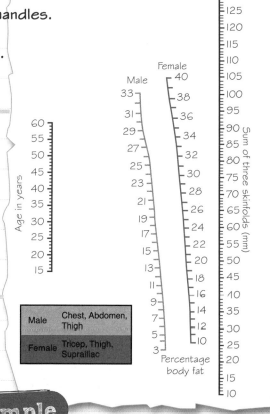

Advantage: an accurate test of body fat.

Disadvantages: can be uncomfortable; the subject may need to readjust clothing which can be embarrassing.

Body fat percentage results for ages 16–29:

| Rating | Males | Females |
|---|---|---|
| Very low | <7 | <13 |
| Slim | 7–12 | 13–20 |
| Ideal | 13–17 | 21–25 |
| Overweight | 18–28 | 26–32 |
| Obese | 29+ | 33+ |

## Worked example

Simon is 24 years old and has a total skinfold measurement of 74 mm.

What is his percentage body fat?   **(1 mark)**

His percentage body fat would be 20 per cent.

## Now try this

Tabita is 17 years old and has a body fat percentage of 23 per cent.

What is the total sum of her skinfold measurements?   **(1 mark)**

# Fitness tests: body mass index (body composition 2)

Body mass index (BMI) is one test used to measure body composition.

## Characteristics of body mass index testing

- Measures: whether weight is appropriate to height
- Units: kg/m²
- Equipment: measuring scales and a tape measure

## Method

1. Measure your body weight in kilograms.
2. Measure your height in metres.
3. Use the formula:

$$\frac{\text{BODY WEIGHT (kg)}}{\text{HEIGHT (m)} \times \text{HEIGHT (m)}}$$

Practice makes perfect – make sure you can remember and use the calculation to predict BMI, it will not be given to you in the test.

### Validity

BMI is not always an accurate measure of body composition for elite sports performers as it does not take muscle mass into account. Muscle is heavier than fat and therefore a muscular athlete like a weightlifter with very little body fat could be considered obese according to BMI calculations.

Advantages: the test is simple, quick and needs no specialised equipment.

Disadvantage: it is not always accurate for muscular individuals.

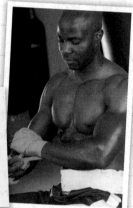

BMI is not the best way of testing the body composition of a muscular individual, such as the boxer in this image.

### Interpreting results

If Ben is 1.6 m tall and weighs 62 kg his BMI would be:

$$\frac{62}{1.6 \times 1.6} = 24 \, \text{kg/m}^2$$

Looking at the table below, this means that he is a healthy weight for his height.

| Rating | BMI (kg/m²) |
|---|---|
| Underweight | <19 |
| Desirable | 20–25 |
| Overweight | 26–30 |
| Obese | 31+ |

Make sure you **learn** the formula for BMI.

## Worked example

Give one advantage of BMI testing over skinfold testing. **(1 mark)**

BMI testing does not need any specialised equipment. You need skinfold callipers for skinfold testing.

## Now try this

Luke is a javelin thrower. He is 1.8 m tall and weighs 102 kg.

**(a)** Calculate his BMI. **(1 mark)**

**(b)** Using the information provided in the table above and, considering Luke's sport, interpret his result. **(2 marks)**

# Fitness tests: bioelectrical impedance analysis (body composition 3)

Bioelectrical impedance analysis is one test used to measure body composition.

## Characteristics of bioelectrical impedance analysis

Bioelectrical impedance analysis measures the resistance encountered by a small electrical current passed through your body.

- Measures: percentage body fat
- Equipment: bioelectrical impedance analysis machine, alcohol pads, weighing scales, tape measure and electrodes
- How it works: fat-free mass lets the current pass through your body more easily, therefore the higher the resistance the higher the body fat.

Advantage: you only have to uncover the left hand and foot so it is less embarrassing than the skinfold test.

Disadvantages: the equipment is expensive; it relies on the subject being well hydrated and not having done any vigorous exercise 12 hours prior to the test; having eaten or just woken up can also impact test scores.

## Method

1. Remove the sock and shoe on the left foot.
2. Lie the subject down on a flat surface, preferably a mat or bed.
3. Wipe their left foot with an alcohol wipe.
4. Move left hand and foot away from body.
5. Place electrodes on the left hand and foot.
6. The test passes a small electrical current through the body and a score is recorded on the analyser.

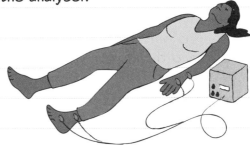

## Reliability

The reliability of this test is compromised if the person being tested is not properly hydrated. Dehydration can result in a higher body fat reading.

Always read the answers carefully – eating **before** the test should be avoided but that's not what option C says!

## Worked example

Name **three** methods that can be used to estimate body composition. **(3 marks)**

Body mass index (BMI), skinfold callipers and bioelectrical impedance analysis.

During the online test, if you want to know how long you have left you can click the 'time' button.

## Now try this

Which **two** of the following factors may reduce the reliability of bioelectrical impedance analysis? **(2 marks)**

A ☐ Exercising before the test

B ☐ Sleeping before the test

C ☐ Eating after the test

D ☐ Drinking before the test

E ☐ Drinking after the test

# Fitness tests: muscular endurance – abdominal

Fitness tests can be used to assess muscular endurance. The SIT-UP TEST is used to measure LOCALISED muscular endurance in the abdominal area.

## Characteristics of the sit-up test

- Measures: endurance of the abdominal muscles
- Units: reps/minute
- Equipment: exercise mat and a stopwatch

## Method

1. Perform a warm-up. Lie on the mat with your knees bent and your feet flat on the floor. Your feet can be held by a partner if required.

2. Fold your arms across your body.

3. Use an assistant to time you for 1 minute. Complete as many full sit-ups as you can in this time.

4. A full sit-up is one where you raise yourself up to 90° and then lower yourself back to the floor.

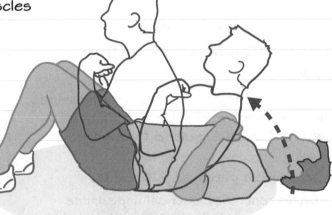

Performing the 1-minute sit-up test.

## Interpreting results

| Rating | Males | Females |
|---|---|---|
| Excellent | 49–59 | 42–54 |
| Good | 43–48 | 36–41 |
| Above average | 39–42 | 32–35 |
| Average | 35–38 | 28–31 |
| Below average | 31–34 | 24–27 |
| Poor | 25–30 | 18–23 |
| Very poor | 11–24 | 3–17 |

## Reliability

To ensure the test is reliable it is important that the same warm-up is completed each time the test is conducted.

Advantages: it is easy to conduct and doesn't need lots of equipment.

Disadvantages: it is easier if you have someone to help you and it is not suitable for people with back injuries.

### Worked example

Which of the following is a test of muscular endurance?          **(1 mark)**

A ☐ Skinfold testing

B ☐ Sit and reach test

C ☑ 1-minute sit-up test

D ☐ Grip dynamometer test

If unsure of the answer in multiple-choice questions, look critically at each individual answer.

Think about how things like the use of a partner can impact on results.

### Now try this

Gerry completes the sit-up test. The first time his friend holds his feet, the second time he completes the test on his own.

Identify **one** impact of this change in method.
          **(1 mark)**

# Fitness tests: muscular endurance – upper body

Fitness tests can be used to assess muscular endurance. The PRESS-UP TEST is used to measure LOCALISED muscular endurance in the upper body.

## Characteristics of the press-up test

- Measures: endurance of the muscles in the upper body
- Units: reps/minute
- Equipment: exercise mat and a stopwatch

## Method

1. Take up a full press-up position on the mat. Your arms should be fully extended.

2. Use an assistant to time you for 1 minute. Complete as many full press-ups as you can in this time.

3. A full press-up is one where the elbows are bent to 90° and then fully extended.

## Interpreting results

| Rating | Males (reps/minute) | Females (reps/minute) |
|---|---|---|
| Excellent | 45+ | 34+ |
| Good | 35–44 | 17–33 |
| Average | 20–34 | 6–16 |
| Poor | <19 | <5 |

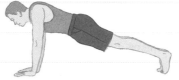
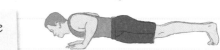

Performing the 1-minute press-up test.

## Modified press-ups

A slightly less challenging version of the test can be done in a bent knee position. Beginners might prefer this version.

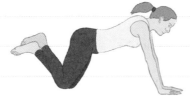

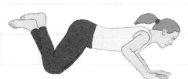

Alternative press-up position with knees bent.

## Interpreting test results of modified press-ups

| Rating | Number of reps |
|---|---|
| Excellent | 39+ |
| Good | 34–38 |
| Average | 17–33 |
| Fair | 6–16 |
| Poor | <6 |

Look at the following data.

Using the tables above, decide what each person's score tells you about their level of upper body muscular endurance. Fill in the final column of the table below with the correct rating. **(4 marks)**

| Name | Test | Score | Rating |
|---|---|---|---|
| Sally | Modified | 32 | Average |
| Imran | Standard | 47 | Excellent |
| James | Standard | 17 | Poor |
| Ceri | Standard | 33 | Good |

## Reliability and validity

To ensure the results are valid, make sure you take note of what kind of press-ups have been completed. To ensure reliability the test conditions should be the same every time test is completed. For example, completing all tests indoors.

Why would this test **not** be an appropriate measure of abdominal endurance? **(1 mark)**

# Fitness tests: speed – 35 m sprint test

Fitness tests can be used to measure speed. A performer's speed can be measured using the 35 m sprint test.

## Characteristics of the 35 m sprint test

- Measures: sprint speed
- Used by: sprinters, long jumpers, footballers
- Units: seconds (s)
- Equipment: two cones, tape measure, stopwatch, flat non-slip surface in excess of 45 m long

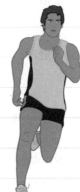

Advantages: requires minimal equipment; is easy to set up; can be conducted inside or outside.

Disadvantage: you might need another person to help with the test.

## Method

1. Allow performers to complete a warm up.
2. Measure out a 35 m straight line using a measuring tape.
3. Mark either end with cones.
4. Take up the sprint start position at one end.
5. On the timer's command, sprint to the other cone.
6. The stopwatch is stopped when your torso crosses the line.
7. Conduct the test three times with a 3 minute recovery between each test.
8. Take the fastest of the three times as the score.

## Interpreting results

| Rating | Male | Female |
|---|---|---|
| Excellent | <4.8 | <5.3 |
| Good | 4.8–5.09 | 5.3–5.59 |
| Average | 5.10–5.29 | 5.6–5.89 |
| Fair | 5.3–5.6 | 5.9–6.2 |
| Poor | >5.6 | >6.2 |

## Reliability and validity

This is a valid test for speed, however it is a more valid test for a 100 m sprinter than a cyclist as it is a better replication of their sport.

To ensure the test is reliable it must conducted in the same way each time, the 35 m distance should be accurately measured, the same warm-up completed and it should be performed in the same environmental circumstances (terrain, weather, incline).

### Worked example

Clara and Aadil both score 5.5 in a 35 m sprint test.

Who has the better sprint speed relative to their gender?   **(1 mark)**

```
Clara as she would be rated as
good. Aadil would only be rated
as fair.
```

### Now try this

Imagine you were sprinting in a sports hall and then in a field. What would make the experiences different? Why might it be easier in a sports hall?

Fatima wants to use the 35 m sprint test to measure improvements in speed as a result of training. The first test was conducted in a sports hall and the second on a field.

Give **two** examples of how reliability may have been compromised.   **(2 marks)**

# Fitness tests: multistage fitness test (MSFT) (aerobic endurance 1)

Fitness tests can be used to assess aerobic endurance. The multistage fitness test (MSFT) assesses aerobic fitness by predicting maximum oxygen uptake. This is also known as the bleep test.

## Characteristics of the multistage fitness test (MSFT)

- Measures: your predicted maximum oxygen uptake (aerobic endurance). (See page 1 to remind yourself of its definition.)
- Equipment: a flat non-slip surface, a 30 m tape measure, cones, the MSFT CD, a CD player, someone to record the results

## Method

1. Allow performers to complete a warm-up. Using the tape to measure, place two cones 20 m apart on a flat surface.

2. Line up on the start line. After the triple beep, run slowly to the other cone. You must reach the other cone before the next beep.

3. After the beep, run back to the other cone. Do not get ahead of the beeps.

4. As the beeps get closer together, you will need to run faster.

5. Keep running until you are physically exhausted or have failed to reach the cone by the time the beep has sounded three times.

6. Record the level and shuttle that you reached. Use this information to predict your $VO_2$ max.

> Advantages: the test is easy to conduct and can be done both indoors and outside; you can also test lots of people at once.
>
> Disadvantage: you must have a copy of the MSFT CD.

## Oxygen intake

$VO_2$ max is the maximum amount of oxygen a person's body is able to take in and use. It is measured in ml/kg/min and is the best measure of aerobic endurance.

## Reliability and validity

The reliability of this test relies on the distance being accurately measured every time and on the environment the test is conducted in remaining constant. The test is more valid for a long-distance runner than a long-distance swimmer as it more closely reflects their activity.

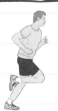

> Performing the multistage fitness test.

← 20 metres →

> For 'discuss' questions always make sure you consider all sides of the question. Make a plan for extended answer questions so that you make sure you cover everything.

## Worked example

> What is the unit of measurement for aerobic fitness? **(1 mark)**
>
> A ☐ mm/kg/min　　B ☐ ml/mg/min
>
> C ☑ ml/kg/min　　D ☐ Kgm/s

## Now try this

A coach organises for his football team to undertake the multistage fitness test to measure the team's aerobic endurance.

> Discuss the advantages and disadvantages of the multistage fitness test for the football coach.
> **(8 marks)**

# Fitness tests: forestry step test (aerobic endurance 2)

Fitness tests can be used to assess aerobic endurance. You need to know about the forestry step test, which is a modified version of the Harvard step test and is used as a fitness test for the police and fire service.

## Characteristics of the test

- Measures: aerobic endurance/$VO_2$ max
- Equipment: a step bench – 40 cm high for males and 33 cm high for females, a metronome set at 90 beats per minute (22.5 steps per minute), a stopwatch

## Method

1. Record body weight in clothing.
2. Stand directly opposite the bench and start stepping in time with the beat of the metronome.
3. As soon as you start stepping, start the stopwatch.
4. Step up and down continuously in time with the beat for 5 minutes.
5. After 5 minutes, stop immediately and locate your radial (wrist) pulse.
6. 15 seconds after stopping, count your pulse for 15 seconds and record this number.

## Interpreting results

After obtaining your 15 second pulse, transfer it to the table appropriate for your age and gender. Find your weight in kg and the value where these two scores meet. This is your approximate $VO_2$ max. So, if Daniel has a 15 second pulse of 22 and weighs 63 kg his $VO_2$ max is approximately 63 ml/kg/min.

| Pulse count | Maximal oxygen consumption ($VO_2$ max) | | | |
|---|---|---|---|---|
| 24 | 60 | 60 | 60 | 60 |
| 23 | 62 | 62 | 61 | 61 |
| 22 | 64 | 64 | 63 | 63 |
| 21 | 66 | 66 | 65 | 65 |
| 20 | 68 | 68 | 67 | 67 |
| Weight (kg) | 54.5 | 59.1 | 63.6 | 68.2 |

Forestry step test aerobic fitness values for males.

Advantages: this test is easy to perform and needs little equipment; it can be self-administered.

Disadvantage: some people might not have the fitness or coordination to keep stepping for 5 minutes.

## Reliability

Help ensure reliability by measuring the height of the step and making sure the pulse is taken at the correct time.

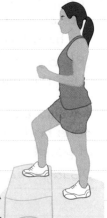

Performing the forestry step test.

33 cm

This question has **two** marks – ensure you define the term and give the unit of measurement to get both marks.

Define $VO_2$ max and give the unit of measurement used. **(2 marks)**

The maximum amount of oxygen an athlete is able to take up and use effectively. It is measured in ml/kg/min.

Identify **two** reasons why a PE teacher might choose the forestry step rather than MSFT to measure the aerobic endurance of their class. **(2 marks)**

# Fitness tests: Illinois agility run test (agility)

Fitness tests can be used to assess agility. The Illinois agility run test measures speed and agility.

## Characteristics of the Illinois agility run test

- Measures: speed and agility
- Used by: rugby players and netball players
- Units: seconds (s)
- Equipment: tape measure, stopwatch and eight cones

Advantages: can be set up anywhere on a non-slip surface and requires minimal equipment.

Disadvantage: needs someone to help with timing.

## Remember

Make sure you can remember how to define agility. Remind yourself on page 6.

## Reliability

It is really important that the distances between cones are accurately measured every time the test is conducted to ensure that the course remains exactly the same.

## Method

1. Lie face down by the start cone.
2. On 'go', get up and run around the course, following the red line, as quickly as possible.
3. The stopwatch is stopped and your time recorded when you pass the finish cone.

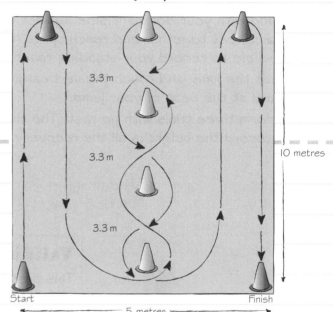

There is a specific layout for the Illinois agility test.

## Interpreting results

| Gender | Excellent | Above average | Average | Below average | Poor |
|--------|-----------|---------------|---------|---------------|------|
| Male | <15.2 | 15.2–16.1 | 16.2–18.1 | 18.2–19.3 | >19.3 |
| Female | <17.0 | 17.0–17.9 | 18.0–21.7 | 21.8–23.0 | >23.0 |

The Illinois agility run test results (in seconds).

## Worked example

Bahiya is a 17-year-old hockey player. She completes the Illinois agility run test in 17.3 seconds.

What does this tell us about her agility? **(1 mark)**

A ☐ It is average    B ☐ It is below average

C ☐ It is poor    D ☑ It is above average

## Now try this

Why is it important to accurately measure out the Illinois agility run course each time the test is conducted? **(1 mark)**

Think about the reliability of test results when answering this question.

# Fitness tests: vertical jump test (anaerobic power)

Fitness tests, such as the vertical jump test, can be used to assess anaerobic power.

## Characteristics of the vertical jump test

- Measures: anaerobic power in the legs
- Units: kgm/s

## Method

1. Perform a short warm-up before starting.
2. Stand with your dominant side against the board, feet together and reach up as high as possible to record your standing reach height.
3. Make the jump and touch the vertical jump board at the peak of your jump.
4. Perform three trials with no rest. The time taken to record the height is all the recovery needed.

## Interpreting results

| Rating | Males (kgm/s) | Females (kgm/s) |
|---|---|---|
| Above average | >105 | >90 |
| Average | 95 | 80 |
| Below average | <85 | <70 |

Advantages: minimal equipment required; simple to set up and conduct; the test can be done in almost any setting.

Disadvantages: can't be conducted on your own – someone needs to take the measurement; technique plays a part in maximising the score.

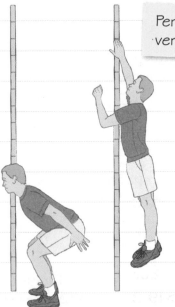

Performing the vertical jump test.

## Validity and reliability

This test is a valid measure of anaerobic power in the legs; it would not be a valid measure of anaerobic power in any other body part. To ensure reliability each time the test is completed it should be:
- conducted at the same time of day
- conducted after the same warm-up
- conducted in the same conditions (inside, outside, surface)
- measurements should be taken by the same person using a metre rule or a vertical jump measuring board.

## Worked example

What does the vertical jump test measure?

A ☐ Anaerobic power in the arms

B ☑ Anaerobic power in the legs

C ☐ Agility in the legs

D ☐ General fitness

Think about the motion you go through when performing the test.

## Now try this

Tomas decides to conduct the vertical jump test. Tomas knows how tall he is so he marks his height on the wall in his garden and decides to work out the readings from there using a ruler. He doesn't warm up and after one jump he takes the reading and finishes the test. The next day, he completes the test in the gym at school using a metre ruler.

Identify **one** problem with the reliability of Tomas' vertical jump test result. **(1 mark)**

# Fitness tests: grip dynamometer (strength)

Fitness tests can be used to measure strength. The grip dynamometer test measures the strength of the grip-squeezing muscles of the hand.

## Characteristics of the grip dynamometer test

- Measures: strength of the grip-squeezing muscles of the hand
- Units: KgW
- Equipment: a spring device – a grip dynamometer
- How it works: When force is applied, the spring in the dynamometer is compressed and the needle moves, indicating the result.

## Method

1. Adjust the handgrip size so the dynamometer is comfortable.
2. Stand up, with your arms by the side of your body.
3. Hold the dynamometer parallel to side of your body, with the display facing away from you.
4. Squeeze as hard as possible for 5 seconds, without moving your arm.
5. Carry out three trials on each hand, with a 1 minute rest between trials.

## Interpreting results

| Rating | Males aged 15–19 years (KgW) | Females aged 15–19 years (KgW) |
|---|---|---|
| Excellent | >52 | >32 |
| Good | 47–51 | 28–31 |
| Average | 44–46 | 25–27 |
| Below average | 39–43 | 20–24 |
| Poor | <39 | <20 |

Advantages: easy to use; can be conducted anywhere; doesn't need much equipment; is fast to complete.
Disadvantages: equipment is specialised; can only test one person at a time as expensive to buy multiple dynamometers.

## Validity

Think carefully about WHY you are doing a particular fitness test. The grip dynamometer test would not be a suitable test to determine the leg strength of a sprinter.

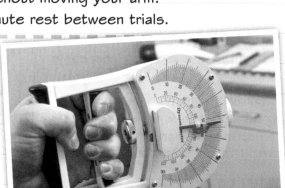

You must remember to use the same hand each time so the result is reliable.

## Worked example

Antoni gets a score of 42 KgW in the grip dynamometer test.

Using the table above, what does this tell you about his grip strength?
**(1 mark)**

It tells you that his grip strength is below average.

## Now try this

Alice scores 22 KgW in the grip dynamometer test.

What fitness training method would be most appropriate to help her improve this score?

A ☐ Continuous training

B ☐ Weight training

C ☐ Circuit training

D ☐ Flexibility training

# Fitness tests: sit and reach test (flexibility)

Fitness tests can be used to assess flexibility. The sit and reach test measures flexibility in a LOCALISED area: the lower back and hamstrings.

## Characteristics of the sit and reach test

- Measures: flexibility in the lower back and hamstrings
- Used by: gymnasts and hurdlers
- Units: cm or inches

## Method

1. Use a sit and reach box.
2. Remove shoes and sit with straight legs and feet flat against the box.
3. In a slow, steady movement, stretch and reach as far forward as possible, sliding your hands on top of the box. Keep your knees straight throughout.
4. Record distance reached.

Advantage: it is quick and easy to do.

Disadvantage: variations in trunk and arm length can make comparisons hard.

### Remember

Many fitness tests are specific. Make sure you know exactly what they are measuring. For example, the sit and reach test would not help you measure shoulder flexibility so when answering questions about it make sure all of your response is relevant.

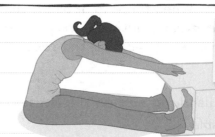

Performing the sit and reach test.

### Remember

PROTOCOL is another way of saying how a test is carried out (the method).

### Reliability

You need to make sure that you have the same length and type of warm-up each time you do the test as warming up may increase flexibility.

## Interpreting results

The table below shows the data for the sit and reach test for 16–19-year-olds. Where do you think you would fit in? What does this say about your flexibility?

| Gender | Excellent | Above average | Average | Below average | Poor |
|--------|-----------|---------------|---------|---------------|------|
| Male | >14 | 14.0–11.0 | 10.9–7.0 | 6.9–4.0 | <4 |
| Female | >15 | 15.0–12.0 | 11.9–7.0 | 6.9–4.0 | <4 |

Sit and reach test results (in cm).

## Worked example

Annika has a sit and reach test score of 5.5 cm.

Explain what this information tells us about her shoulder flexibility. **(2 marks)**

```
It would tell us nothing about her shoulder
flexibility as the sit and reach test is
a measurement of the flexibility of the
hamstrings and muscles of the lower back.
```

Remember that many fitness tests are specific and apply to particular localised areas of the body.

## Now try this

Explain why you think a hurdler's score in the sit and reach test would be high. **(2 marks)**

# Exam skills 1

The onscreen test for Unit 1 lasts one hour and includes a variety of question types. There will be questions on ALL the learning aims: A, B and C. You can answer the questions in any order.

## Practise

✓ The more you revise the more you will understand.

✓ Complete as many practice questions as you can prior to the exam.

✓ Practise all of the different types of question.

✓ Practise marking questions too – it will help you to see what the question is asking.

## Answering multiple-choice questions

✓ Read the question carefully.

✓ Look out for the KEY WORDS in the question.

✓ Read all the options carefully.

✓ Rule out any answers that you know are wrong.

✓ Read the CONTEXT of the question – look for the most appropriate answer.

✓ Select the most appropriate answer for the context.

---

### Worked example

Maja plays netball.

Which of the following tests is **least** relevant to her sport?
**(1 mark)**

A ☐ Illinois agility run test
B ☐ 35 m sprint test
C ☐ Vertical jump test
D ☑ Sit and reach test

This question is asking you to identify the test which is **least appropriate** for the performer. You need to consider the aspects of fitness that you think this performer would use and see if there are tests that measure these.

**Option A** tests agility and this would be very useful for a netball player who needs to dodge and change direction quickly.

**Option B** tests speed which is also helpful.

**Option C** tests anaerobic power in the legs which would be useful to a netball player who needs to jump high to make interceptions.

**Option D** measures flexibility which, out of all of the options, would be the least relevant to a netball player – and therefore is the correct answer.

---

### Worked example

Which of these statements about fartlek training is **not** correct?
**(1 mark)**

A ☐ Fartlek training means 'speed play' in Swedish

B ☐ Fartlek training is continuous but with changes of pace

C ☑ Fartlek training contains periods of work and rest

D ☐ Fartlek training is used by team sports players (e.g. basketball/volleyball)

The question is asking you to identify the statement which is **not** correct. First check to see if any of the options are obviously about fartlek training.

**Option A** is a definition of fartlek training so this option can be discounted.

Out of the remaining options, **B** and **D** are correct as fartlek training is used by team sports players and closely mimics the fitness requirements of a team sport.

As we know that **options B** and **D** are correct, we know that **C** is the incorrect answer as there are no periods of rest in fartlek training – just periods of lower intensity work.

43

# Exam skills 2

It is important to familiarise yourself with the features of the online test.

TIME: this shows/hides the time that has elapsed since the start of the test. Find it at the bottom right of your screen.

HELP: this tells you about the features of the test and the tools available. It does not provide technical help. If you have a technical problem in the online test then tell the invigilator straight away.

ACCESSIBILITY PANEL: if you are struggling to read the screen, try adjusting the colours or magnifying the screen.

NEXT: this moves the test on to the next question.

WORKING BOX: use the working box for rough notes or calculations at any time.

CALCULATOR: use this when you have to carry out any calculations.

REVIEW: this button lets you go back through the test and check your answers. Any questions you 'flagged' show on this screen.

FLAG: you can do the questions in any order. If one puzzles you, leave it and carry on. Use the Flag button to mark it, so you won't forget about it.

PREVIOUS: this moves the test back to the previous question.

QUIT: when you click this button a pop-up window asks if you want to quit the test. Answer 'yes' or 'no'. If you press 'no' you return to the question you were answering. When you have finished and checked all your answers use this button.

## Answering short-answer questions

Some questions will require you to write shorter answers to show your understanding. Most short-answer questions will be worth 1, 2 or 3 marks each.

- ✓ Read the question carefully.
- ✓ Look out for the key words.
- ✓ Look at the number of marks available for the question.
- ✓ Make sure you make the same number of statements as there are marks available. For example, if the question is worth 3 marks, make at least three statements.
- ✓ Try not to repeat the question in your answer.
- ✓ If the question relates to a particular activity then make sure you make reference to it in your answer.
- ✓ Make sure you look at the key command word – have you been asked to describe, explain or discuss?

Show the difference by describing one term and then the other. These are important terms to know.

Make sure your answer is specific to rugby.

## Worked example

Describe the difference between reliability and validity in relation to fitness testing. **(2 marks)**

Validity refers to whether a test actually measures what it says it measures. Reliability is about whether the test can be repeated and the same accurate results collected.

## Worked example

Explain why a high level of agility is beneficial for a rugby player. **(2 marks)**

A high level of agility is important for a rugby player because they need to be able to dodge the opposition in order to keep hold of the ball and avoid being tackled. If they have good agility they will be quicker and more able to change direction at speeds which will allow them to avoid players on the other team.

# Exam skills 3

Learn how to spot the different COMMAND words used in questions. Command words tell you exactly what sort of answer is needed.

## Key command words

Describe: give a description of...

State: list or name what the question is asking for.

Outline: briefly list the main features.

Identify: select one option or name something.

Explain: give reasons why something is as it is.

Justify: provide reasons why something is valid or why you chose something.

Compare: identify and explain the similarities and differences.

Discuss: give reasons or present facts and explain their impact on the topic.

Summarise: give an account of the main points.

Interpret: make a judgement about something.

## Worked example

Describe the key features of PNF (proprioceptive neuromuscular facilitation) and how it is carried out.
**(4 marks)**

PNF is used to develop mobility, flexibility and strength. It is performed against the resistance of a partner or immoveable object. The performer stretches their muscle to the upper limit and then contracts the muscle isometrically for 6–10 seconds. This is then followed by a passive stretch.

Note that this question is worth 4 marks. After writing the answer read it through to check that it is correct and contains enough information.

The command word in this question is 'describe'. This means you need to say how PNF is used, and detail how it is carried out.

## Preparation

It is really important that you prepare well for your test, both in the weeks and days before.

### Pace yourself

- ✓ Think about how you learn best – mind maps, tape recordings, posters, etc. Create materials that will suit you.
- ✓ Try to peak at the right time – this means planning your revision.
- ✓ Don't leave revision too late – plan well in advance.
- ✓ Try to find a time and a place where you work best – try to avoid distractions.
- ✓ Make sure you leave time for other things – being organised is key.

### Checklist for the day

- ✓ Get up in plenty of time – don't be rushed.
- ✓ Eat well.
- ✓ Get there early.
- ✓ Make sure you know how long you have in the exam.
- ✓ Work out how long you can spend on each question.
- ✓ Check the spelling in your answers.
- ✓ Don't panic!

# Major voluntary muscles 1

Knowing the location and actions of major VOLUNTARY MUSCLES is really important for both sports performers and people working in the sport and active leisure industry. Voluntary muscles are dealt with in more detail on page 50. Make sure you know the locations of the main voluntary muscles and their roles.

## Biceps and triceps

Name: BICEPS

Location: Front of the upper arm

Role: FLEXION at the end of the elbow

Example: Upwards phase of a biceps curl

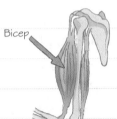
Bicep

FLEXION means bending a joint.

Name: TRICEPS

Location: Back of the upper arm

Role: EXTENSION of the arm at the elbow

Example: Straightening the arms in a chest press

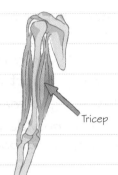
Tricep

EXTENSION means straightening a joint.

## Quadriceps and hamstrings

Name: QUADRICEPS

Location: Front of the upper leg

Role: Extension of the leg at the knee

Example: Straightening the leading leg going over a hurdle

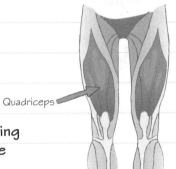
Quadriceps

Name: HAMSTRINGS

Location: Back of the upper leg

Role: Flexion of the leg at the knee

Example: Bending the trailing leg going over a hurdle

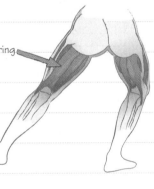
Hamstring

## Worked example

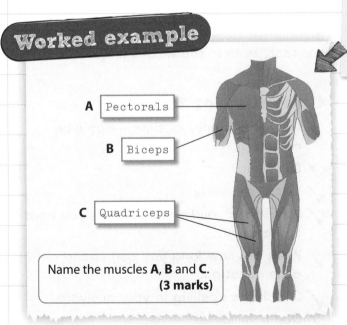

A  Pectorals

B  Biceps

C  Quadriceps

Name the muscles **A**, **B** and **C**.
**(3 marks)**

When writing the names of muscles, make sure that you use the full name. For example, you should always write 'quadriceps' rather than 'quads'.

## Now try this

Complete the blanks by identifying the muscles and their roles.   **(4 marks)**

The muscles found at the back of the upper legs are the _____. Their role is _____ of the legs at the knees.

The muscles found at the front of the upper legs are the _____. Their role is _____ at the knees.

# Major voluntary muscles 2

Make sure that you know the location of these muscles, and their roles, and can give examples of their use.

## Trapezius, latissimus dorsi and erector spinae

Name: TRAPEZIUS
Location: Upper back, from the neck across the shoulders
Role: Neck extension and shoulder elevation
Example: The butterfly arm action in swimming – when the arms are thrown sideways and backwards out of the water

Name: LATISSIMUS DORSI
Location: Side of the back
Role: ADDUCTS the upper arm at the shoulder/rotates the humerus
Example: Bringing arms back to the sides during a straight jump in trampolining

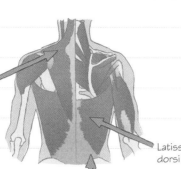

Trapezius
Latissimus dorsi
Erector spinae

Name: ERECTOR SPINAE
Location: Runs either side of the spine
Role: Extension of the spine
Example: This muscle is used during a back extension – you lie flat on your front with your arms by your side and raise your shoulders off the floor so that you are arching backwards

> ADDUCTS means to move towards the midline of the body.

## Pectorals, obliques and abdominals

Name: PECTORALS
Location: Front of the upper chest
Role: Adducts the arm at the shoulder
Example: Follow-through from a forehand drive in tennis

Name: ABDOMINALS
Location: Front of the torso, below the upper chest
Role: Flexion and rotation of the spine
Example: Pike diving position

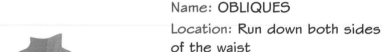

Pectorals
Obliques
Abdominals

Name: OBLIQUES
Location: Run down both sides of the waist
Role: Lateral (sideways) flexion of the spine
Example: Oblique curls – these involve bending over to one side of the body without leaning forwards or backwards and then returning to upright

## Worked example

The image shows a client exercising using a weights machine.

Which muscle is being contracted to allow him to pull the bar down? **(1 mark)**

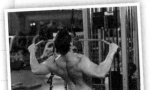

A ☐ Pectorals
B ☐ Abdominals
C ☑ Latissimus dorsi
D ☐ Obliques

If you are unsure which muscle is responsible for a movement, try performing the movement and see if you can feel which muscle is moving.

## Now try this

Choose words from the box below to complete the following sentences on the location of the major voluntary muscles. **(3 marks)**

The pectorals are found at the front of the _____ and are important when doing press-ups. The abdominals are found below the _____ and allow flexion of the trunk. The obliques are found at the _____ of the waist and allow sideways flexion of the trunk.

| | | |
|---|---|---|
| trapezius | chest | back |
| neck | pectorals | side |

# Major voluntary muscles 3

Make sure that you know the location of these muscles, and their roles, and can give examples of their use.

## Gluteus maximus, gastrocnemius, deltoid and soleus

Name: GLUTEUS MAXIMUS

Location: The largest muscle in the buttocks

Role: Extension of the leg at the hip

Example: Lifting the leg back at the hip when running

Name: GASTROCNEMIUS

Location: Back of the lower leg

Role: Pointing toes (i.e. PLANTARFLEXION of the ankle) – extension at the ankle

Example: Pointing toes when performing a straddle jump in trampolining

Name: DELTOID

Location: The top of the shoulder

Role:
- ABDUCTS the arm at the shoulder
- Shoulder flexion and extension

In combination this is CIRCUMDUCTION

Examples:
- Lifting your arms above your head to block the ball in volleyball
- Rotating your arm during the bowling action in cricket

Name: SOLEUS

Location: Beneath the gastrocnemius

Role: Plantarflexion of the ankle with knee bent

Example: Pushing off from the blocks in a sprint start

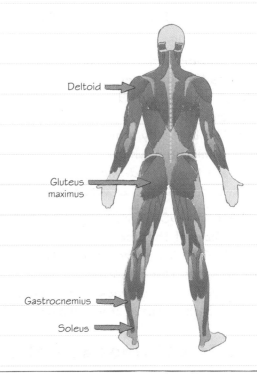

ABDUCTS means to move away from the midline of the body – see page 68.

## Remember

Always use the correct name for the gastrocnemius, not the calf. Remember it has a 'C' sound in it

Gast ... roC  nem ... ius.

---

## Worked example

Which muscle group is responsible for raising the dumb-bells out to the side?   **(1 mark)**

**A** ☐ Biceps

**B** ☐ Gluteus maximus

**C** ☑ Deltoids

**D** ☐ Soleus

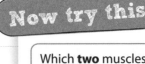

## Now try this

Which **two** muscles are responsible for plantarflexion of the ankle while pushing off the blocks in a sprint start?   **(2 marks)**

**A** ☐ Gluteus maximus

**B** ☐ Soleus

**C** ☐ Deltoid

**D** ☐ Gastrocnemius

**E** ☐ Trapezius

# Types of muscle

There are three different types of muscles found within the human body.

 **Voluntary muscle**

- Also known as SKELETAL or STRIATED muscle.
- Location: attached to the skeleton.
- Characteristics:
  - under conscious control (i.e. you have to make them move)
  - responsible for body movements.

 **Involuntary muscle**

- Also known as SMOOTH or VISCERAL muscle.
- Location: found in the stomach, intestines and blood vessels (i.e. veins and arteries).
- Characteristics:
  - controlled unconsciously (i.e. it works automatically to aid things like digestion)
  - slow, rhythmic contractions.

 **Heart muscle**

- Also known as CARDIAC muscle.
- Location: found only in the heart.
- Characteristics:
  - controlled unconsciously (i.e. required to keep heart beating)
  - fairly rapid and sustained contractions to pump blood from the heart to the body tissues.

> Involuntary muscle is found in the stomach, intestines and blood vessels.

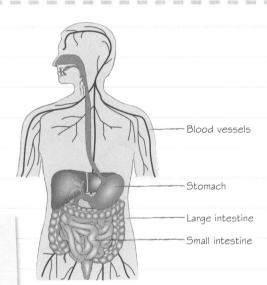

Blood vessels
Stomach
Large intestine
Small intestine

> When answering multiple-choice questions start by ruling out any answers you know are wrong.

**Worked example**

Which of the following is a characteristic of involuntary muscle? **(1 mark)**

A ☐ Contractions are rapid and sustained

B ☑ It is found in the intestines, stomach and blood vessels

C ☐ It is under conscious control

D ☐ It is responsible for body movements

**Now try this**

Using the words from the box below, complete the following sentences. **(5 marks)**

Voluntary muscles, also known as _____ or striated muscles, are attached to the _____. Involuntary muscles, also known as smooth or _____ muscles, are found in the stomach, blood vessels and _____. Cardiac muscle is only found in the _____.

| intestines | skeletal | visceral |
| skeleton | heart | |

# Voluntary muscle movements

There are many muscles in the body. Knowing their location and role is important in all sporting activities.

## Antagonistic pairs

Skeletal muscles work together to provide movement of the joints.

While one muscle CONTRACTS, another RELAXES to create movement.

Muscles working together like this are called ANTAGONISTIC PAIRS.

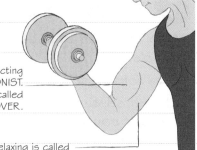

The muscle contracting is the AGONIST. It is sometimes called the PRIME MOVER.

The muscle relaxing is called the ANTAGONIST.

There are four examples of antagonistic muscle pairs on page 51.

## Worked example

The image below shows a sprinter.

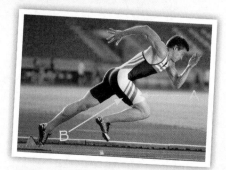

Choose from the words below to describe the muscles at A and B.    **(2 marks)**

antagonist   agonist   involuntary   isometric

**A** is the   antagonist

**B** is the   agonist

## Tendons

Muscles are connected to bones via TENDONS. When the muscles contract, they pull on the tendons which pull on the bones. This creates the movement.

The sprinter needs to **contract** muscle B to push off from the blocks. This muscle is the **agonist** or **prime mover**. In order for this to happen the muscle at A must **relax**. So this muscle is the **antagonist**.

The roles of the two muscles change when the action of the sprinter changes. In the leg that is pushing **down** the roles of the muscles are reversed.

## Now try this

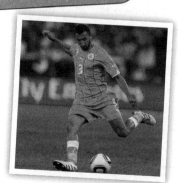

The image shows a footballer kicking a ball.

Using the correct muscles from the box below, fill in the blanks to identify the muscles that are responsible for kicking the ball.    **(2 marks)**

The _____ are the agonist when the striker extends his leg at the knee to strike the football and the _____ are the antagonist.

| quadriceps | hamstrings | abdominals |
| --- | --- | --- |
| latissimus dorsi | obliques | |

# Antagonistic muscle pairs

Antagonistic muscle pairs resist the action of each other. As one muscle CONTRACTS the other RELAXES to help movement. Here are four examples of antagonistic muscle pairs.

 **Biceps and triceps**

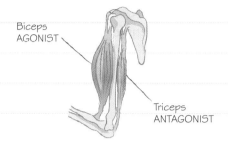

Biceps
AGONIST

Triceps
ANTAGONIST

 **Quadriceps and hamstrings**

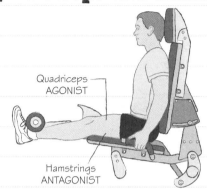

Quadriceps
AGONIST

Hamstrings
ANTAGONIST

 **Rectus abdominis and erector spinae**

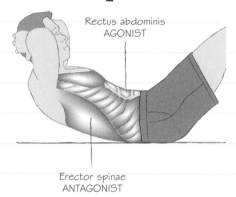

Rectus abdominis
AGONIST

Erector spinae
ANTAGONIST

 **Pectoralis major and trapezius**

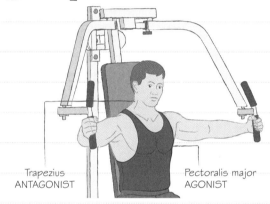

Trapezius
ANTAGONIST

Pectoralis major
AGONIST

## Worked example

Which **one** of the following muscles is contracting to allow the weight trainer to lift the dumb-bell?
**(1 mark)**

A ☑ Bicep

B ☐ Tricep

C ☐ Hamstring

D ☐ Pectoralis

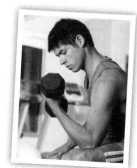

Look closely at the image for a clue to the answer.

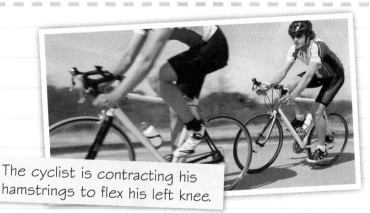

The cyclist is contracting his hamstrings to flex his left knee.

## Now try this

The image shows an athlete sprinting.

Which set of antagonistic muscle pairs is the athlete using the most to generate her speed?
**(2 marks)**

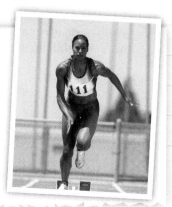

# Types of contraction

There are three type of muscle contraction. You need to know what they are and be able to explain when they are used in sports movements.

 **Concentric contraction**

CONCENTRIC CONTRACTION occurs when the muscle shortens in length and develops tension as it contracts.

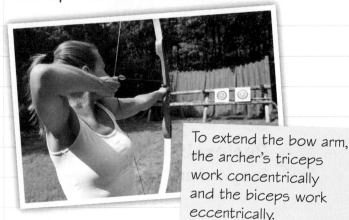

To extend the bow arm, the archer's triceps work concentrically and the biceps work eccentrically.

 **Eccentric contraction**

ECCENTRIC CONTRACTION is the development of tension as the muscle lengthens.

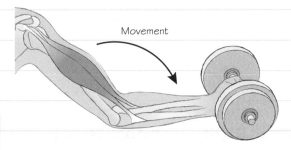

Movement

The biceps muscle is demonstrating eccentric contraction as the dumb-bell is lowered.

**3 Isometric contraction**

ISOMETRIC CONTRACTION is when the muscle contracts, develops tension and stabilises the body, but does not change in length.

The position being held by this gymnast requires isometric contraction of the abdominals, erector spinae, biceps, triceps, deltoids, trapezius, latissimus dorsi and pectoral muscles in his upper body.

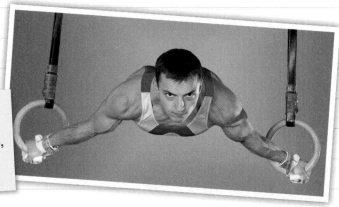

## Worked example

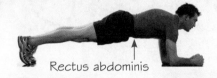

Rectus abdominis

Which muscular contraction is happening at the rectus abdominis during the plank? **(1 mark)**

A ☐ Concentric

B ☐ Eccentric

C ☑ Isometric

D ☐ Standard contraction

## Now try this

1 Which of the following is the correct definition of an isometric muscle contraction? **(1 mark)**

A ☐ When a muscle shortens in length and develops tension

B ☐ When a muscle contracts but does not change in length

C ☐ When a muscle lengthens and develops tension

D ☐ When a muscle lengthens but does not develop tension

2 With reference to a specific muscle (or muscle group) and sporting movement, give **one** example of a concentric contraction. **(1 mark)**

# Slow twitch muscle fibres (type I)

Slow twitch muscle fibres are sometimes called type I muscle fibres. You need to know which types of sporting activities they are important for and why.

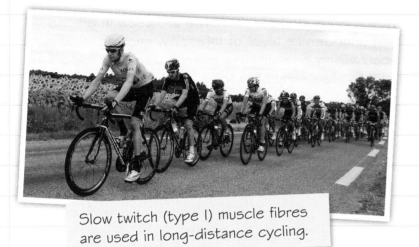

Slow twitch (type I) muscle fibres are used in long-distance cycling.

Slow twitch (type I) muscle fibres are used in endurance sports, such as long-distance cycling and long-distance running events. They are important for athletes like Sir Bradley Wiggins and Mo Farah.

Slow twitch muscle fibres are also used in team sports that last a significant amount of time, for example rugby, hockey and netball.

## Characteristics

Try to learn these five key characteristics.
Slow twitch muscle fibres:

- contract slowly
- produce low amounts of force
- can cope with prolonged activity
- are slow to fatigue
- have a high aerobic capacity.

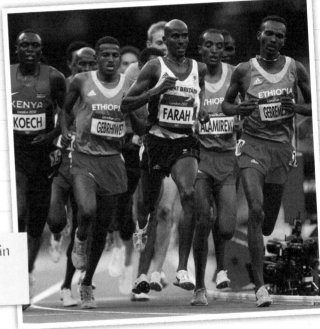

Slow twitch muscle fibres are used in long-distance running because they can cope with prolonged activity.

**Always** check how many items a question is asking you for.

Use the characteristics of muscle fibre types to explain why they are beneficial for a particular activity.

### Worked example

State **one** characteristic of slow twitch (type I) muscle fibres.          **(1 mark)**

They can cope with prolonged activity.

### Now try this

Explain **one** reason why slow twitch (type I) muscle fibres are beneficial for endurance athletes.          **(2 marks)**

# Fast twitch muscle fibres (type IIa)

Fast twitch muscle fibres are sometimes called type IIa muscle fibres. You need to know which kinds of sporting activities they are used in and why.

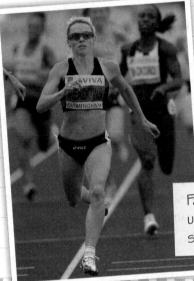

Fast twitch (type IIa) muscle fibres are used in events involving a moderate level of intensity, such as middle-distance running or swimming events. They are important for athletes like Jenny Meadows and Michael Phelps.

Type IIa muscle fibres are also required in racquet sports, particularly during rallies. 400 m, 800 m and 1500 m track events will also need the contribution of type IIa fibres.

Fast twitch (type IIa) muscle fibres are used in moderate intensity events, such as middle-distance running.

## Characteristics

Try to learn these four key characteristics.

Fast twitch muscle fibres (type IIa):

- contract more rapidly than type I (but not as fast as type IIb)
- produce medium amounts of force
- are fairly resistant to fatigue
- have a medium level of aerobic capacity.

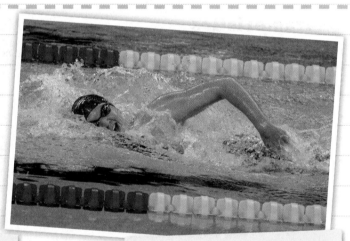

Type IIa muscle fibres help swimmers in long-distance events avoid fatigue.

Link the intensity of an event to the characteristics of the muscle fibre types.

## Worked example

Explain why fast twitch (type IIa) muscle fibres are beneficial for middle-distance runners and swimmers. **(2 marks)**

Both athletes compete in events that require elements of speed over a longer period of time than short sprints. Their muscles need to contract quicker than they would in a long-distance event. Type IIa muscle fibres are also fairly resistant to fatigue. This is important when taking part in a long sprint, as you would not want to fatigue after 200 m.

## Now try this

Which of the following is a characteristic of fast twitch (type IIa) muscle fibres?
**(1 mark)**

A ☐ They produce low amounts of force

B ☐ They fatigue quickly due to lactic acid build-up

C ☐ They are fairly resistant to fatigue

D ☐ They can cope with prolonged activity

# Fast twitch muscle fibres (type IIb)

Fast twitch muscle fibres are sometimes called type IIb muscle fibres. You need to know which kinds of sporting activities they are important for and why.

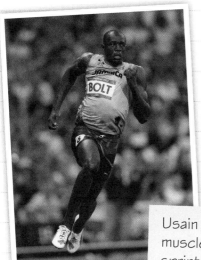

Fast twitch (type IIb) muscle fibres are used in short-distance activities that are high-intensity anaerobic events and require 'all-out' effort, such as 100 m sprints or sprinting for a football. They are important for athletes like Usain Bolt and Cristiano Ronaldo.

Other events that require the use of type IIb muscle fibres are field events in athletics, such as the long jump, high jump, javelin and discus. These fibres are also required for certain actions within sports, such as a jump shot in basketball, a baseball swing and a serve in tennis.

Usain Bolt uses fast twitch (type IIb) muscle fibres in the 100 m and 200 m sprints, which require 'all-out' effort.

## Characteristics

Try to learn these four key characteristics.
Fast twitch muscle fibres (type IIb):

* have the fastest contractions of the three muscle fibre types
* produce the highest amounts of force
* fatigue most quickly due to lactic acid build-up
* produce explosive power.

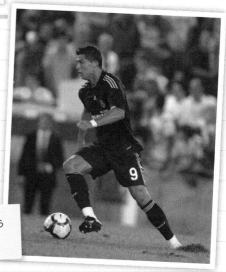

Cristiano Ronaldo uses fast twitch muscle fibres (type IIb) to produce short speed bursts.

## Worked example

Remember to include examples from sport or exercise scenarios if a question asks you to provide an example.

**(a)** State **one** characteristic of a type IIb muscle fibre. **(1 mark)**

Type IIb muscle fibres produce explosive power.

**(b)** Identify **one** sporting event that requires this characteristic. **(1 mark)**

They are used in events that require all-out effort such as the take-off in the high jump.

## Now try this

**(a)** State **one** characteristic of a fast twitch (type IIb) muscle fibre. **(1 mark)**

**(b)** With reference to this characteristic, explain why fast twitch (type IIb) muscle fibres are beneficial for 100 m sprinters. **(2 marks)**

# Recruitment of muscle fibres with varied levels of muscular effort

As the levels of effort required in an activity change, so does the level of muscle fibre type recruitment. The graph below shows how, as a performer increases exercise intensity, a greater number of muscle fibres are used.

## Section A

Low amounts of muscular force (for example, walking slowly) require only slow twitch (type I) muscle fibres. These muscles are recruited first.

## Section B

As the intensity of the activity increases (for example, moving from walking to running), the type and number of muscle fibres changes. As intensity increases, type IIa muscle fibres are added.

## Section C

As the intensity of the activity further increases (for example, from running to sprinting), type IIb muscle fibres are recruited. These fibres are only added once intensity reaches 60+% of the maximum.

Remember that in ramp-like recruitment of muscle fibres, type I are recruited first, followed by type IIa, and type IIb are recruited last.

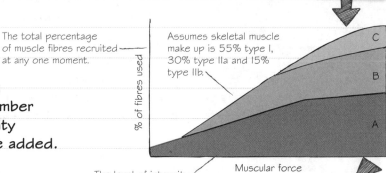

The total percentage of muscle fibres recruited at any one moment.

Assumes skeletal muscle make up is 55% type I, 30% type IIa and 15% type IIb.

% of fibres used

Muscular force

The level of intensity, increasing to the right.

The increased recruitment of muscle fibres as activity increases is known as **ramp-like recruitment** of muscle fibres.

---

Think about the number of marks available. Marks can be awarded for an explanation of how muscular force links with the percentage of fibres recruited. Provide an example that demonstrates that you understand how all three fibres can be used during a sporting event.

## Worked example

Explain what is meant by 'ramp-like recruitment of muscle fibres'. **(2 marks)**

Ramp-like recruitment of muscle fibres means that as the intensity of the activity increases, the type and number of muscle fibres will change. Type I are recruited first at low intensity, followed by type IIa, and type IIb are recruited last at the highest intensity of activity.

---

## Now try this

Tariq is running a 1000 m race. This graph shows his progress.

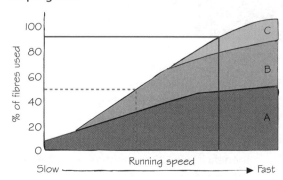

The dashed line suggests a speed that's 50% of Tariq's maximum. This requires 50% of his total muscle fibres to be recruited. Tariq is using type I muscle fibres and some type IIa muscle fibres. The solid line suggests a speed that's 90% of his maximum. This increased effort requires 90% of his total muscle fibres to be recruited. Tariq is now using type IIb muscle fibres.

Explain what this graph tells us about muscle fibre recruitment in a long-distance race.

**(4 marks)**

# Bones of the skeleton

In order to understand how the body works during exercise, you need to know about the bones of the skeleton and where they are located. The skeleton is made up of 205 bones.

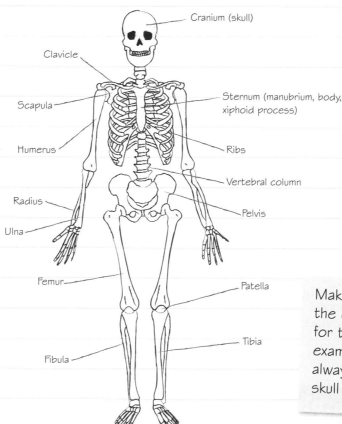

Cranium (skull)

Clavicle

Scapula

Humerus

Radius

Ulna

Femur

Fibula

Sternum (manubrium, body, xiphoid process)

Ribs

Vertebral column

Pelvis

Patella

Tibia

Make sure you learn the correct names for the bones — for example, you should always refer to the skull as the cranium.

## Worked example

Label the bones on the skeleton.
**(3 marks)**

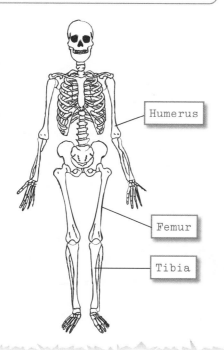

Humerus

Femur

Tibia

Make sure that you know how to spell the names of bones in case the question asks you to write them out, rather than select them from a list.

It's important that you learn the location of all the bones in the diagram above. That information will be a good starting point in questions like this!

## Now try this

Match each of the bones to the correct description.
**(6 marks)**

| Bone | Location |
|------|----------|
| Femur | Smallest bone at the shoulder joint |
| Radius | Smallest bone in the lower leg |
| Ulna | Largest bone in the lower leg |
| Clavicle | Largest bone in the body and leg |
| Fibula | Smallest bone in the forearm |
| Tibia | Largest bone in the forearm |

# Different types of bone

As part of your understanding of the skeleton, you need to know about the five different types of bone.

LONG bones
• Bones that are used in large movements and act as levers
• Often long (some exceptions such as metacarpals and phalanges)
• Often have a tubular structure
• Each end is covered by hyaline (or articular) cartilage
EXAMPLES include the femur and humerus

SHORT bones
• Bones that are used in smaller movements
• Cube-shaped bones
EXAMPLES include the carpals and tarsals

FLAT bones
• Protect internal organs
• Thin, flat and slightly curved
• Have a large surface area
EXAMPLES include the cranium, scapula and sternum

IRREGULAR bones
• Irregular in shape
EXAMPLES include the vertebrae and some facial bones

SESAMOID bones
• Small oval-shaped bones
• Embedded in tendons
• Located where a tendon passes over a joint
EXAMPLES include the patella

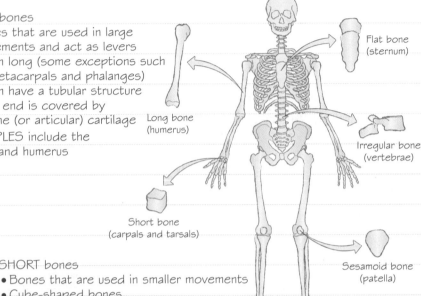

Long bone (humerus)

Flat bone (sternum)

Irregular bone (vertebrae)

Short bone (carpals and tarsals)

Sesamoid bone (patella)

## Worked example

In the table below, give an example and a characteristic of each type of bone.

**(5 marks)**

| Type of bone | Example | Characteristic |
|---|---|---|
| Long | Femur | Each end is covered by articular cartilage |
| Short | Carpals | Cube shaped |
| Flat | Scapula | Has a large surface area |
| Irregular | Vertebrae | Irregular in shape |
| Sesamoid | Patella | Embedded in tendons |

Use a table like this to learn examples. Cover each column or row and test yourself until you can name them all.

## Now try this

Using an example, explain the role of flat bones.    **(2 marks)**

Try to learn examples of each type of bone. If you think about where your example is located it will help you to answer this question.

# The axial and appendicular skeleton

The human skeleton is broken down into two parts: the axial skeleton and the appendicular skeleton. You need to know which bones make up the different parts.

 **The axial skeleton**

The axial skeleton provides support and protection of the organs and a means for the attachment of muscles.

 **The appendicular skeleton**

The appendicular skeleton allows movement and protects some of the major organs. This is also a means for the attachment of muscles.

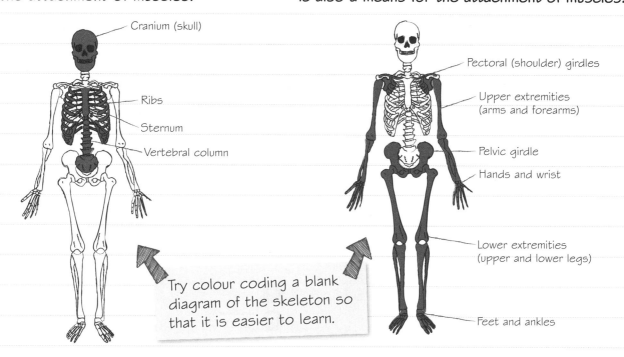

Cranium (skull)
Ribs
Sternum
Vertebral column

Pectoral (shoulder) girdles
Upper extremities (arms and forearms)
Pelvic girdle
Hands and wrist
Lower extremities (upper and lower legs)
Feet and ankles

Try colour coding a blank diagram of the skeleton so that it is easier to learn.

## Worked example

Complete each of the following sentences to show whether the bones are part of the axial or appendicular skeleton. **(4 marks)**

1 The cranium is part of the `axial` skeleton.

2 The shoulder girdle is part of the `appendicular` skeleton.

3 The pelvic girdle is part of the `appendicular` skeleton.

4 The sternum is part of the `axial` skeleton.

## Now try this

Which **one** of the following bones is **not** part of the axial skeleton? **(1 mark)**

A ☐ Cranium

B ☐ Ribs

C ☐ Pelvic girdle

D ☐ Vertebral column

Remember if you want to come back to a question in the onscreen test you can 'flag' it.

# Structure of the rib cage and vertebral column

The RIB CAGE and VERTEBRAL COLUMN provide shape and support for the body, and protection for internal organs. They also allow movement of the body.

## The rib cage

The rib cage is made up of 12 pairs of ribs in total. These can be divided into:

- TRUE RIBS (7 pairs) that attach to the vertebrae and the sternum
- FALSE RIBS (3 pairs) that attach to vertebrae at the back and the rib above at the front
- FLOATING RIBS (2 pairs) that only attach to the vertebrae at the back.

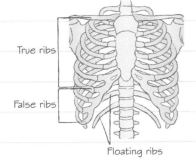

True ribs

False ribs

Floating ribs

## The vertebral column

The vertebral column is:

- made up of 33 vertebrae in total
- separated into FIVE regions as shown in the diagram.

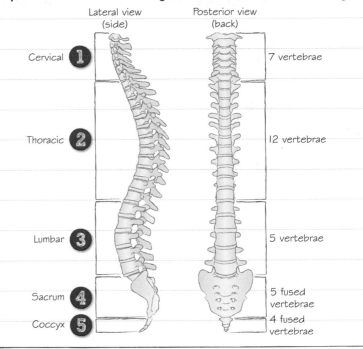

Lateral view (side)   Posterior view (back)

Cervical 1 — 7 vertebrae

Thoracic 2 — 12 vertebrae

Lumbar 3 — 5 vertebrae

Sacrum 4 — 5 fused vertebrae

Coccyx 5 — 4 fused vertebrae

## Importance of the rib cage

The rib cage also plays an important role in breathing by moving upwards and outwards to allow the lungs to expand. It is important in contact sports such as rugby as it protects vital organs.

## Now try this

Label the regions below on the diagram of the vertebral column.   **(5 marks)**

Cervical

Sacrum

Thoracic

Coccyx

Lumbar

To remember all the different parts of the vertebral column it may help to break it down into the five regions. Look at the diagram above.

# Functions of the skeletal system 1

The skeleton has six main functions that are important in sport and exercise. You need to know about the function of the skeletal system in a range of different sporting activities.

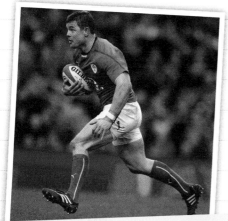

The skeleton provides a rugby player, such as Brian O'Driscoll, with protection.

 **Protection**

The skeleton provides PROTECTION to VITAL ORGANS. For example, a rugby player's:

- rib cage protects their heart and lungs when being tackled
- cranium protects their brain if they fall or if they are tackled illegally
- vertebral column protects their spinal cord.

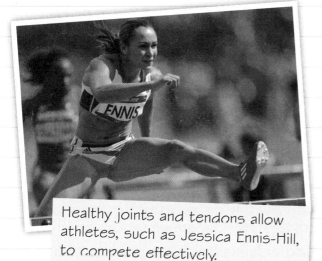

Healthy joints and tendons allow athletes, such as Jessica Ennis-Hill, to compete effectively.

**2 Muscle attachment and movement**

Muscles are attached to bones via tendons. Bones have joints that permit MOVEMENT.

When a muscle contracts, the tendon it is connected to pulls on the bone and produces movement.

The joints between bones permit movement but without healthy MUSCLE ATTACHMENT sites (tendons) and joints, athletes would not be able to compete effectively.

## Worked example

Which of the following options completes the sentence below? **(1 mark)**

The skeletal system protects _____

A ☐ vital organs; for example bones, muscles and tendons

B ☑ by providing a hard structure over the organ needing protection

C ☐ by providing a structure for support

D ☐ by producing red blood cells that fight disease

## Now try this

Explain how **one** function of the skeleton is important for long-jumpers.

**(2 marks)**

When asked to explain a function of the skeleton, make sure that you talk about what it does and give an example, rather than just stating a function.

# Functions of the skeletal system 2

There are four further functions of the skeleton that you need to know about.

 **Support**

Your skeleton provides a FRAMEWORK for your body and therefore SUPPORTS you.

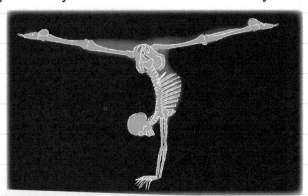

The skeleton provides the support that enables a gymnast to balance when performing a handstand.

 **Shape**

Your skeleton gives you SHAPE. When your skeleton grows as you change from a child to an adult, your shape changes with it.

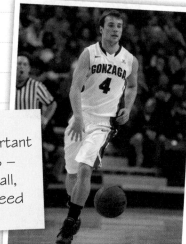

Body shape is particularly important in certain sports – such as basketball, where players need to be tall!

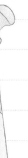 **Blood production**

Red blood cells are produced in the BONE MARROW of long bones. Having more red blood cells means you have the ability to carry more oxygen, which can help sport performance.

Red blood cell production

 **Storage of minerals**

Bones store four minerals:

1. CALCIUM: important for bone and teeth formation, clotting blood and muscle contraction
2. PHOSPHOROUS: important for bone and teeth formation, and energy metabolism
3. SODIUM: important for muscle contraction and nerve impulses
4. POTASSIUM: important for muscle contraction and the functioning of the nervous system.

## Worked example

Always relate your answers to sport to demonstrate your understanding.

List the **six** main functions of the human skeleton. **(6 marks)**

```
1) Protects many vital organs, such as lungs,
heart and brain during sporting activities; 2)
Provides muscle attachment, which aids movement
during all motions such as the long or high
jump; 3) Gives the body shape which affects
what sports you are suited for; 4) Provides
a framework to support the body; 5) Red blood
cell production; 6) Stores minerals.
```

## Now try this

Identify the **four** key minerals that are stored in bones.
**(4 marks)**

# Classifications of joints

As we have already seen, joints allow movement. There are three main classifications of joints.

 **Fixed (immovable) joints**

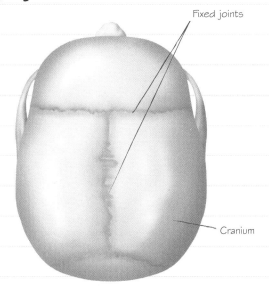

Fixed joints

Cranium

- Don't allow any movement
- Examples: joints of the skull and sacrum
- Important for protection

 **Slightly moveable (cartilaginous) joints**

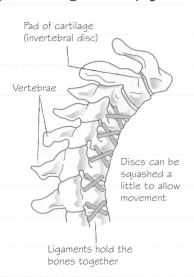

Pad of cartilage (invertebral disc)

Vertebrae

Discs can be squashed a little to allow movement

Ligaments hold the bones together

- Allow only slight movement
- Examples: joints between vertebrae in the spine

**3 Freely moveable (synovial) joints**

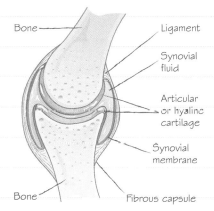

Bone — Ligament
Synovial fluid
Articular or hyaline cartilage
Synovial membrane
Bone — Fibrous capsule

- Have the greatest range of movement
- Example: knee joint
- Used in most sporting actions
- There are SIX different types of synovial joints (see page 64).

see page 64

## Worked example

Fill in the blanks to complete the sentence.
**(2 marks)**

A | fixed | or | immovable | joint does not allow any movement.

Note that each of the different classifications of joints has **two** names. It is good to know both names for each classification of joint.

## Now try this

Which **one** of the following classifications of joint allows the greatest range of movement?
**(1 mark)**

A ☐ Fixed

B ☐ Cartilaginous

C ☐ Synovial

D ☐ Immovable

# Types of freely moveable joints

Freely moveable joints (also known as synovial joints) can be divided into the following types based on the type of movement that they permit.

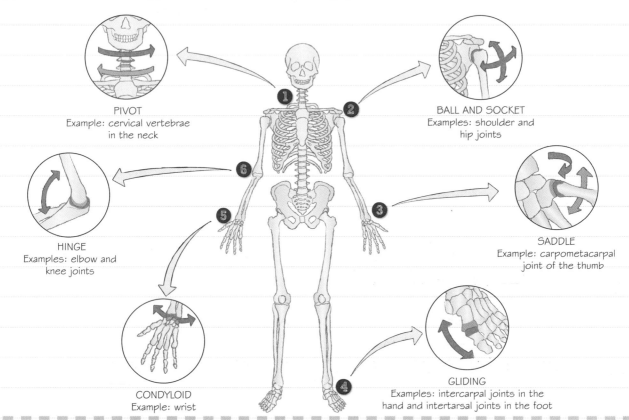

PIVOT
Example: cervical vertebrae in the neck

BALL AND SOCKET
Examples: shoulder and hip joints

HINGE
Examples: elbow and knee joints

SADDLE
Example: carpometacarpal joint of the thumb

CONDYLOID
Example: wrist

GLIDING
Examples: intercarpal joints in the hand and intertarsal joints in the foot

## Worked example

One example of a ball and socket joint is the shoulder.

Which **one** of the following joints is another example of a ball and socket joint? **(1 mark)**

A ☐ Elbow      B ☐ Knee

C ☐ Wrist      D ☑ Hip

In the onscreen test, choose the answer that you think is correct and then click on the box next to it.

## Now try this

Try labelling a blank skeleton until you can name all the joints.

Fill in the blanks to complete the sentences. **(3 marks)**

1 The carpometacarpal joint of the thumb is an example of a _____ joint.

2 The cervical vertebrae are an example of a _____ joint.

3 The knee joint is an example of a _____ joint.

# Types of cartilage

Cartilage is a strong, flexible connective tissue found in various parts of the body, including joints. There are three different types of cartilage in the body: FIBROCARTILAGE, HYALINE (or ARTICULAR) cartilage and ELASTIC cartilage. You need to know the location and functions of each type.

 **Fibrocartilage**

- Found in tendons
- Also found in intervertebral discs of the vertebral column
- Contains collagen fibres
- It is tough and acts as a shock absorber

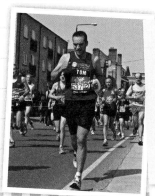

Fibrocartilage helps to protect a marathon runner's spine when they are doing lengthy road running. It absorbs the repetitive shock that happens with every running step on the road.

## ② Hyaline (or articular) cartilage

- Found on the articulating surface of bones
- Helps to ensure smooth joint movement by reducing friction between the bones
- Protects bones in the joint from wear and tear
- Acts as a shock absorber and absorbs stress
- Provides support – it is tough, flexible tissue that supports your weight when you move (e.g. when you run)

Hyaline cartilage is also found in the trachea and bronchi.

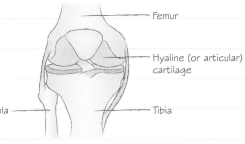

Femur

Hyaline (or articular) cartilage

Fibula

Tibia

## ③ Elastic cartilage

- Flexible tissue that gives support in a number of places (e.g. the ear and epiglottis)
- Found in the external part of the ear and the epiglottis

Remember to think about how the properties of the cartilage benefit sport performance.

### Worked example

Which type of cartilage is important for protecting a performer's knee joints during the triple jump landing phases?
**(1 mark)**

A ✓ Hyaline (or articular)
B ☐ Elastic
C ☐ Fibrocartilage
D ☐ Collagen fibres

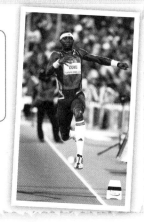

### Now try this

Basketball places lots of stress on a player's knee joints.

Explain how **one** property of hyaline (or articular) cartilage helps to reduce the risk of damage to the knee joints. **(2 marks)**

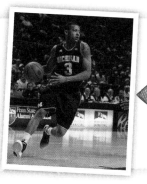

Remember to explain the property first and then explain how it helps to reduce the risk of damage.

# Synovial joint structure

All synovial joints contain the elements listed below. You need to know the structure of a synovial joint to help you understand how the joint works.

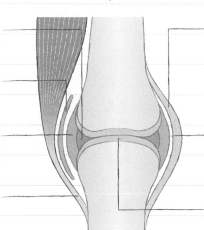

SYNOVIAL FLUID
Fills the joint capsule and lubricates and nourishes the joint.

BURSA
A fluid–filled sac between the tendon and the bone that helps to reduce friction.

JOINT SYNOVIAL CAPSULE
Encases the joint and comprises the synovial membrane and fibrous capsule. Helps to protect the joint.

TENDON
White fibrous cords of connective tissue that attach muscle to bone. Made of collagen, so they are tough and strong. Found towards the end of muscle tissue.

LIGAMENT
Tough connective tissue that joins bone to bone and holds the bones together. Made up of tough, tightly packed elastic fibres that can withstand sudden stresses and provide strength to prevent injuries, such as dislocations.

SYNOVIAL MEMBRANE
Acts as a lining for the joint capsule and produces synovial fluid which lubricates the joint.

BONE ENDS
Covered with slippery hyaline (or articular) cartilage to allow the bones to move smoothly with little friction.

## Worked example

Match the structure to the description provided. **(2 marks)**

Synovial fluid — Lubricates and nourishes the joint

Ligament — Made up of tough, tightly packed elastic fibres

Bone end — Covered with slippery hyaline (or articular) cartilage

Bursa — A fluid-filled sac

> You need to learn the names of the synovial joint structures. Try covering up the labels on the above diagram and try to name each part of the joint.

## Now try this

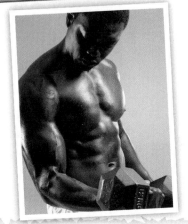

The image shows an example of a synovial joint in action while weight training.

Complete the following statements about the structure of a synovial joint.
**(2 marks)**

1 Tissues that join bone to bone and hold together bones that form a joint are called _____.

2 The fluid-filled sac between the tendon and the bone that helps to reduce friction is called the _____.

# Joint movements 1

Understanding joint movements is central to successful sport performance. You need to know the range of movements that joints can go through and how they relate to actions performed in different sporting activities.

## Joint action: flexion

FLEXION is the term given when the angle at a joint DECREASES.

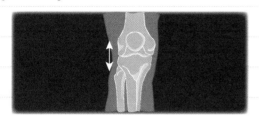

This happens when the bones forming the joint move closer together.

## Joint type and application

FLEXION occurs at hinge joints and ball and socket joints; for example, at the knee when a player is preparing to kick a football.

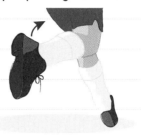

The lower part of your leg gets closer to the upper part of your leg as the angle at the joint decreases.

## Joint action: extension

EXTENSION is the term given when the angle at a joint INCREASES.

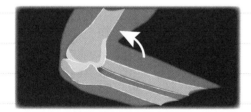

This happens when the bones forming the joint move away from each other.

> If a question asks you about the 'range of movement', make sure that you include both **flexion** and **extension** in your answer as a joint has to move through them both for it to be a **range of movement**.

## Joint type and application

EXTENSION occurs at hinge joints and ball and socket joints; for example, at the knee when following through after kicking a football.

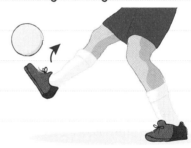

The lower part of your leg gets further away from the upper part of your leg as the angle at the joint increases.

## Worked example

What is the range of movement permitted at a hinge joint, such as the elbow?    **(1 mark)**

The range of movement at the elbow joint is flexion to extension.

## Now try this

State the range of movement that the knee joint has gone through to allow the volleyball player to straighten his leg.

**(1 mark)**

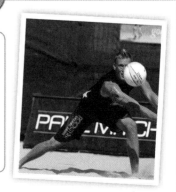

# Joint movements 2

Some other joint movements that occur at ball and socket joints are described below. You need to know about all these.

## Joint actions

ABDUCTION = the movement of a limb AWAY from the midline of the body.

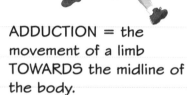

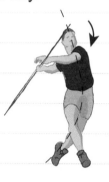

ADDUCTION = the movement of a limb TOWARDS the midline of the body.

ROTATION = when the bone at a joint moves around its own axis, so making a circular movement. Rotation is the movement along a single axis.

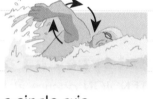

CIRCUMDUCTION = a circular movement of a joint. It is a combination of flexion, extension, abduction and adduction. For example, circumduction occurs when bowling a cricket ball.

Circumduction is really a combination of all of the other joint actions and allows for the biggest range of movement.

## Joint type and application

Abduction occurs at ball and socket joints (hip and shoulder); for example, at the shoulder when reaching out sideways to intercept a netball.

> **Remember**
> If something is 'abducted', it is taken away.

Adduction occurs at ball and socket joints (hip and shoulder); for example, at the hip in the cross-over leg action when throwing a javelin. The leg comes back toward the midline of the body.

> **Remember**
> Adduction starts with 'add' so it is when a limb is added to the midline of the body.

Rotation occurs at ball and socket joints (hip and shoulder), for example at the shoulder when swimming front crawl. The arm rotates around in a circular motion.

## Worked example

Which joint movement is necessary in the right arm of the player with the ball to complete a 'no-look' pass? **(1 mark)**

A ✓ Abduction
B ☐ Adduction
C ☐ Circumduction
D ☐ Rotation

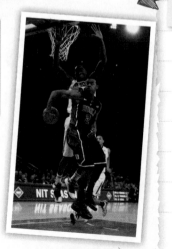

Think about the name for the movement pattern as it will give you a clue to the answer. For example, 'abduct' means to take something away, which suggests movement away from the body.

## Now try this

Choose the correct joint movement from the box below to complete the following sentence. **(1 mark)**

_____ is the movement of a limb towards the midline of the body.

| Abduction | Adduction | Circumduction |
| Flexion | Rotation | |

# Joint movements 3

Other joint movements that you need to know about and understand include PLANTARFLEXION, DORSIFLEXFION, ELEVATION and DEPRESSION.

## Joint action: plantarflexion and dorsiflexion

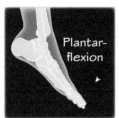

PLANTARFLEXION: bending the foot downwards away from the tibia

DORSIFLEXION: bending the foot upwards towards the tibia

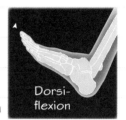

## Joint type and application

Plantarflexion and dorsiflexion occur at the ankle.

For example, plantarflexion occurs when striking a football with the instep.

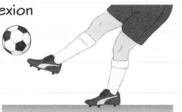

Dorsiflexion occurs, for example, when bending the foot upwards to trap a football with the sole of your boot.

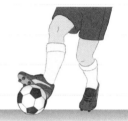

## Joint action: elevation and depression

ELEVATION: upward movement of a part of the body

DEPRESSION: downward movement of a part of the body

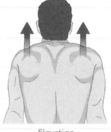 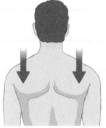

Elevation      Depression

## Joint type and application

Elevation and depression occur at the shoulder joint.

For example, the upward phase in a weightlifting exercise in the gym is elevation and the downward phase is depression.

### Worked example

What is the range of movement permitted at the ankle joint? **(1 mark)**

Dorsiflexion to plantarflexion

If you need to answer a question like this, make sure that you include both **dorsiflexion** and **plantarflexion** in your answer as a joint has to move through them both for it to be a **range of movement**.

### Now try this

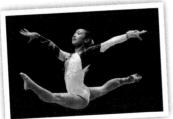

Gymnasts' ankles go through a range of movement when performing leaps and jumps as part of a floor routine.

What range of movement has this gymnast's ankle joints gone through to allow her to point her toes fully? **(1 mark)**

If you struggle with this question try starting the movement and look at your ankle joint.

# Joint movement and muscle group contractions related to sports performance

You need to be able to analyse sports movements by identifying which joints are moving, the range of movements that they are going through and which muscles are involved.

## Analysing Cristiano Ronaldo's volley

Biceps flex the arm at the elbow

Hamstrings flex the leg at the knee

Gastrocnemius plantarflexes the ankle and assists the hamstrings in flexing the leg at the knee

Deltoids abduct the shoulder

Soleus plantarflexes the ankle when the knee is in flexion

Erector spinae extends the spine

Gluteus maximus extends the leg at the hip

## Analysing Tom Daley's pike dive

Trapezius elevates the shoulder

Pectorals flex the arm horizontally

Deltoids flex the shoulder

Quadriceps extend the legs at the knee and assist in hip flexion

Triceps extend the arm

Gastrocnemius plantarflexes the ankle

Abdominals and obliques flex the spine

## Now try this

During the service action, a tennis player's joints go through a range of movements.

Identify which joints are moving, the range of movement they are going through, and analyse how the joints and muscles are interacting.

(8 marks)

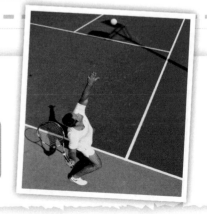

# Structure of the heart

The heart is the central part of the cardiovascular (or circulatory) system, which transports oxygen around the body. It is important to understand the structure of the heart in order to understand the effects of short-term and long-term exercise on it.

## Structure of the heart

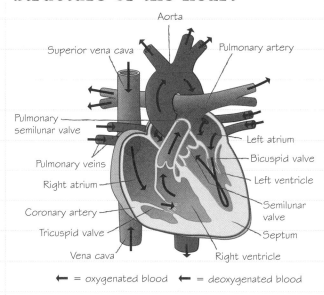

Aorta
Superior vena cava
Pulmonary artery
Pulmonary semilunar valve
Pulmonary veins
Left atrium
Bicuspid valve
Right atrium
Left ventricle
Coronary artery
Semilunar valve
Tricuspid valve
Septum
Vena cava
Right ventricle

⬅ = oxygenated blood    ⬅ = deoxygenated blood

| | |
|---|---|
| Atria | Collect blood |
| Ventricles | Pump blood from the heart |
| Valves | Prevent blood flowing backwards |
| Septum | Separates the two sides of the heart |
| Coronary artery | Supplies heart muscle with oxygenated blood |
| Pulmonary artery | Carries deoxygenated blood to the lungs to allow it to be re-oxygenated |
| Pulmonary veins | Carries oxygenated blood back to the heart from the lungs |
| Aorta | Carries oxygenated blood away from the heart (left ventricle) towards the rest of the body |
| Vena cava | Carries deoxygenated blood back into the heart (right atrium) from the body |

## Worked example

Match each structure below to the correct definition of its function.
**(3 marks)**

**Structure**          **Function**

Valve          Separates the two sides of the heart

Septum          Supplies the heart muscle with oxygenated blood

Coronary artery          Prevents backflow of blood

You need to know the names of the structures of the heart and their functions. Try covering up one column in the table above and write out the missing names or functions.

## Now try this

Label the structures below on the diagram.     **(5 marks)**

| Aorta | Left atrium | Tricuspid valve | Right ventricle | Semi-lunar valve |

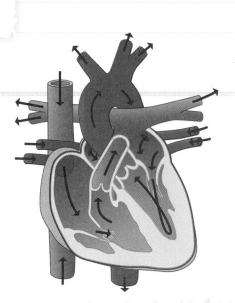

# Types of blood vessels

Blood and the vessels it flows through are also important parts of the cardiovascular/circulatory system. The different types of blood vessels that you need to know are described below.

## Arteries and arterioles

- ARTERIES carry OXYGENATED blood AWAY from the heart – *except the pulmonary artery*, which carries de-oxygenated blood from the heart to the lungs.
- They have THICK, MUSCULAR, ELASTIC WALLS.
- They also have a small internal diameter so that blood flows under HIGH PRESSURE.
- ARTERIOLES connect arteries to capillaries (see below).

## Veins and venules

- VEINS carry DE-OXYGENATED blood from the body to the heart – *except the pulmonary veins*, which carry oxygenated blood from the lungs back to the heart.
- They have THIN WALLS.
- They have a larger internal diameter to allow blood to flow under LOW PRESSURE.
- VALVES in veins prevent backflow of blood, helping VENOUS RETURN.
- VENULES are small veins that connect capillaries to veins.

## Capillaries

- CAPILLARIES are the smallest blood vessels – only one cell thick.
- They connect arterioles to venules.
- Oxygen, carbon dioxide, nutrients and waste products are exchanged through the capillary walls.

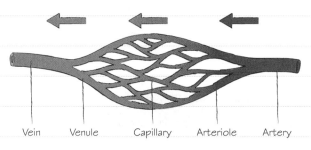

Vein    Venule    Capillary    Arteriole    Artery

## Structure and function

There are lots of differences between the structure and functions of arteries and veins.

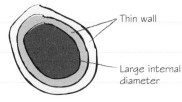

Thick, muscular, elastic wall

Small internal diameter

Artery cross-section

Thin wall

Large internal diameter

Vein cross-section

## Worked example

Describe **one** characteristic of a vein that differs from the structure of an artery.
**(2 marks)**

Veins have a large internal diameter to allow blood to flow through them at a lower pressure, whereas arteries have a smaller internal diameter.

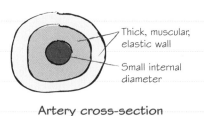

When asked to describe the difference between two structures, make sure that you use words like '**whereas**' or '**however**' to link the two parts of a sentence together and demonstrate that you are trying to show a difference.

## Now try this

Fill in the blanks to explain how capillaries assist in blood flow from arteries to veins. **(2 marks)**

Capillaries carry blood from arteries to veins by connecting
_____ and _____.

# Functions of the cardiovascular system

The cardiovascular system has four main functions, which are important when taking part in sporting activities. You need to know what they are.

 **Circulation and transport**

Blood CIRCULATES and TRANSPORTS CARBON DIOXIDE and other waste products away from the vital organs and muscles.

Carbon dioxide is a waste product created during RESPIRATION (see page 75).

OXYGEN is transported in red blood cells to vital organs and muscles.

Oxygen is needed to produce energy in the muscles.

The cardiovascular system also provides cells with nutrients and transports hormones to cells and organs.

 **Protection**

White blood cells play a major role in PROTECTING the body and keeping us fit and healthy.

They fight INFECTIONS and DISEASES by producing antibodies that destroy any harmful microorganisms that invade the body.

 **Clotting**

The cardiovascular system can also prevent the body from losing too much blood following an injury.

Specialised blood cells, called platelets, form a clot and seal the cut or damaged area. They help to prevent further blood loss or bacteria entering the cut.

 **Temperature regulation**

Blood helps to maintain a constant body temperature of 37°C.

The blood absorbs heat created by internal organs and transports it around the body to maintain the internal temperature.

### What blood is made of

Blood is made up of:
- red blood cells – which carry oxygen
- white blood cells – which protect the body from infection
- platelets – which are involved in clotting
- plasma – a clear fluid that carries nutrients, carbon dioxide and other waste.

## Worked example

Identify **three** substances that are transported in the blood. **(3 marks)**

Oxygen, nutrients and carbon dioxide.

> Make sure that you pay attention to key words and details in the onscreen test questions, such as the number of elements that you are asked to identify, describe etc. in your answer.

## Now try this

Fill in the blanks in the sentence below. **(3 marks)**

If we cut ourselves, our blood _____ to prevent further blood _____ and _____ the cut.

# Functions of the cardiovascular system – thermoregulation

The human body tries to maintain a constant internal temperature of 37°C. You need to know how the skin, blood and circulatory system help with this process through thermoregulation.

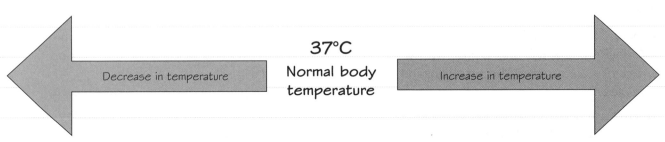

Decrease in temperature

37°C
Normal body temperature

Increase in temperature

For example, due to cold weather

For example, due to warm weather or exercise

## The body's response to cold

The SKIN and SUBCUTANEOUS FAT give insulatory benefits and the body responds to a decrease in temperature in two ways:

1. VASOCONSTRICTION – arterioles (blood vessels) under the surface of the skin narrow (CONSTRICT) so that blood no longer flows through the blood vessels under the skin so little heat is lost through RADIATION

2. SHIVERING – muscle contraction generates heat causing an increase in body heat.

## The body's response to heat

The body responds to an increase in temperature in two ways:

1. VASODILATION – arterioles close to the skin's surface widen (DILATE) therefore increasing the amount of blood flow through the arteriole. Increased blood flow through these blood vessels near the surface of the skin will allow greater heat loss via radiation.

2. SWEATING – sweat glands produce sweat that EVAPORATES from the skin causing heat to be lost.

## Worked example

The body tries to maintain a constant internal temperature of 37°C. The cardiovascular/circulatory system helps maintain a constant temperature through vasoconstriction and vasodilation.

Explain the role of vasodilation in thermoregulation. **(2 marks)**

> During thermoregulation, vasodilation causes the arterioles close to the skin's surface to widen. This increases blood flow through the blood vessels close to the skin's surface so more heat is lost through radiation.

To explain the role of something, you need to say what it does and expand your answer to say how it does it.

## Now try this

The body tries to maintain a constant internal temperature of 37°C. The cardiovascular/circulatory system helps maintain a constant temperature through vasoconstriction and vasodilation.

Explain the role of vasoconstriction in thermoregulation. **(2 marks)**

# Structure of the respiratory system

Muscles need oxygen to function, which is provided through RESPIRATION. To understand this process, you need to know about the structure and functions of the respiratory system. See pages 76 and 77 for more information on its functions.

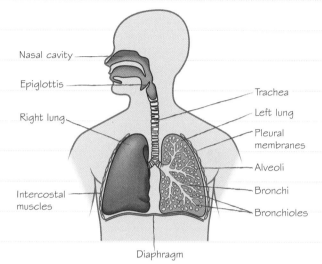

Nasal cavity
Epiglottis
Right lung
Intercostal muscles
Diaphragm
Trachea
Left lung
Pleural membranes
Alveoli
Bronchi
Bronchioles

## Gaseous exchange

Oxygen passes from the alveoli into the blood by diffusion to be circulated around the body. Carbon dioxide is then removed from the blood by gaseous exchange so it can be breathed out. See page 77 for more information about gaseous exchange.

| Structure | Description | Function |
|---|---|---|
| NASAL CAVITY (nose) | Lined with cilia and a mucous membrane | Inhales, moistens, warms and filters air |
| TRACHEA | Tube strengthened by rings of cartilage to prevent collapse | Takes air from the larynx into the bronchi |
| BRONCHI | Two smaller tubes leading to each lung and the bronchioles | Carries air to the lungs |
| ALVEOLI | Small sacs at the end of the bronchioles | Where GASEOUS EXCHANGE takes place |
| PLEURAL MEMBRANES | Line the lungs and thoracic cavity | Pleural fluid between the membranes lubricates the movement of the lungs and prevents damage |

## Now try this

Label the below parts of the respiratory system on the diagram. **(4 marks)**

Trachea    Intercostal muscles

Alveoli    Bronchi

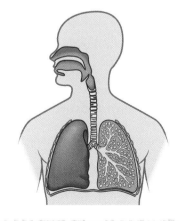

# Functions of the respiratory system 1

In order to get oxygen to the muscles for energy, we need to breathe. Breathing in is referred to as INSPIRATION and breathing out as EXPIRATION.

## Inspiration (the process of breathing in)

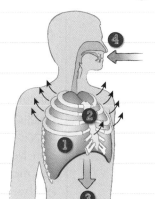

**1** External INTERCOSTAL MUSCLES contract, raising and expanding the ribcage

**2** DIAPHRAGM contracts downwards, increasing the size of the thoracic cavity, allowing the lungs to expand further

**3** Lung volume increases and pressure inside the chest decreases, causing air to rush into the lungs

**4** Air is inhaled

## Expiration (the process of breathing out)

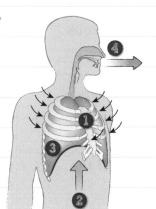

**1** Internal INTERCOSTAL MUSCLES contract, lowering the ribcage

**2** DIAPHRAGM relaxes and pushes up into a dome-shaped position

**3** Lung volume decreases, so pressure inside the chest increases, causing air to be forced out of the lungs

**4** Air is exhaled

## Worked example

Fill in the blanks to complete the description of inspiration. **(5 marks)**

The external intercostal muscles `contract`.

The rib cage `expands`. The diaphragm `contracts` downwards and increases the size of the thoracic cavity. The volume of the lungs `increases` and pressure inside the chest `decreases` causing air to rush into the lungs.

When asked to describe or explain a process such as inspiration, make sure that you break it down into each individual part of the process.

## Now try this

Explain the role of the internal intercostal muscles in expiration. **(2 marks)**

# Functions of the respiratory system 2

GASEOUS EXCHANGE is the process by which oxygen that is breathed in passes into the blood and carbon dioxide is removed from the blood to be expired. It is important that you understand this process.

## Gaseous exchange

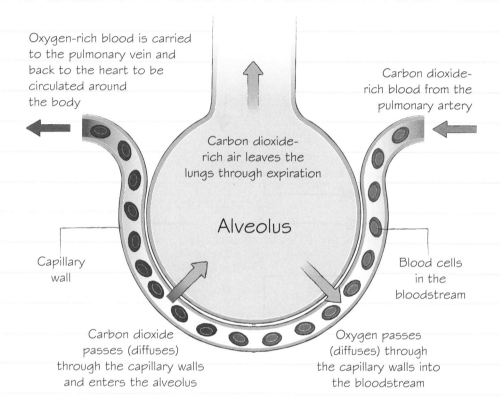

Oxygen-rich blood is carried to the pulmonary vein and back to the heart to be circulated around the body

Carbon dioxide-rich blood from the pulmonary artery

Carbon dioxide-rich air leaves the lungs through expiration

Alveolus

Capillary wall

Blood cells in the bloodstream

Carbon dioxide passes (diffuses) through the capillary walls and enters the alveolus

Oxygen passes (diffuses) through the capillary walls into the bloodstream

---

### Worked example

Identify **two** key parts of gaseous exchange.          **(2 marks)**

    1 Oxygen passing into the blood
    2 Carbon dioxide being removed
      from the blood

### Now try this

Explain the process of gaseous exchange.
**(4 marks)**

If you are asked to 'explain' the process of something, ensure you cover all the steps involved.

# Functions of the cardiorespiratory system

The cardiovascular system and respiratory system work together to help us take part in sport. You need to know their combined functions.

## Blood flow through the heart, body and lungs

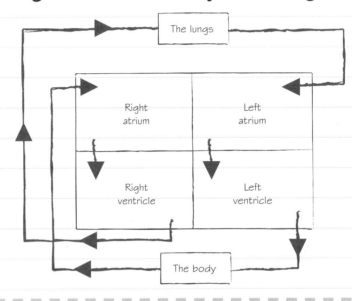

## Other functions

- Supplying oxygenated blood to body tissues
- 'Taking up' oxygen into the body in order to produce energy
- 'Unloading' carbon dioxide, a waste product of respiration, from the body

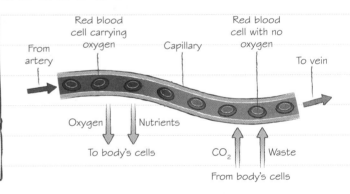

Look at page 72 to remind yourself of the structure of the heart. Ensure you learn it for the test!

Remember you can check the 'time' button throughout the online test to see how long you have left.

## Worked example

Which blood vessel transports blood from the heart to the lungs?          **(1 mark)**

Pulmonary artery

## Now try this

Fill in the blanks below to show how blood is pumped from the heart to the lungs so that it can be re-oxygenated.          **(3 marks)**

The _____ valve opens, your _____ contracts and blood is forced into the _____ to travel to the lungs.

# Exam skills 1

You will have 1 hour to complete the onscreen test. The test is worth 50 marks and will contain a variety of questions, including some multiple-choice questions.

## Answering multiple-choice questions

- ✓ Make a note of the key words in the question.
- ✓ Read all the options carefully.
- ✓ Rule out of the ones you know are wrong.
- ✓ Select what you think is the right answer.
- ✓ Double check the remaining options as well to make sure you are right.

## Choosing the best answers

You need to be really careful when you are choosing your answers. There are often choices that look sensible, but aren't suitable for the CONTEXT of the question.

Always read the question carefully and choose the MOST APPROPRIATE options for the context.

## Worked example

Which **one** of the following is a function of the cardiovascular system?  **(1 mark)**

A ☐ Inspiration
B ☑ Transporting oxygen
C ☐ Support
D ☐ Gaseous exchange

The question is asking you to find the most relevant option for the **cardiovascular** system.

**Options A** and **D** relate to the respiratory system, and **option C** relates to the skeletal system. Therefore **option B** is the correct answer.

The question is asking which muscle group is responsible for **flexing** the leg at the **knee**. You can rule out **options A** and **D** immediately as the deltoids are in the shoulder and the pectorals are in the chest so cannot be involved with flexing the leg at the knee. **Options B** and **C** are both in the upper leg, so could be possible. However, in order to flex the leg at the knee when preparing to kick a football, you have to bring the lower leg backwards and upwards from the knee joint. This means it must be a muscle group at the back of the leg that creates this action as muscles pull (not push), so you can rule out **option B** as the quadriceps are at the front of the leg. As a result, the correct answer is **option C**.

## Worked example

When preparing to kick a football, which of the following muscle groups flexes the leg at the knee?  **(1 mark)**

A ☐ Deltoids
B ☐ Quadriceps
C ☑ Hamstrings
D ☐ Pectorals

# Exam skills 2

As well as multiple-choice questions, you will also have to answer some short-answer questions.

## Answering short-answer questions

✓ Read the question carefully.

✓ Take note of key words.

✓ Note the number of marks available for the question.

✓ Make sure you make the same number of statements as there are marks available. For example, if the question is worth 2 marks, make at least two statements.

✓ Don't repeat words from the question. If you do, make sure you go on to explain in further detail using other words too.

✓ If an activity is referred to in the question, make sure your answers relate to this activity.

✓ Give a range of answers that cover different sports or activities. For example, if you are asked to look at the role of the different muscle fibres in sport, try to look at a range of different sports that best demonstrate the contribution of the different muscle fibres.

✓ The space provided for your answer will be a box where you can write as much as you want – remember to be detailed but concise.

✓ Ensure you use sport- or exercise-related examples as much as possible.

## Identify vs explain

Different questions have different command words. If a question asks you to IDENTIFY, it is asking for a simple statement, but if you are asked to EXPLAIN then make sure your answer is developed and that you give more than a simple statement. You should be using words like BECAUSE or THEREFORE leading you to a more in-depth answer.

## Worked example

Explain **one** characteristic of a fast twitch type IIb muscle fibre and how this benefits a specific sport performance.  **(2 marks)**

One characteristic of a fast twitch type IIb muscle fibre is that it produces a high amount of force, therefore it can produce a high amount of explosive power. This is important in sports events, such as the 100 m sprint, because explosive power is needed to push away from the blocks quickly to allow you to get the best start.

This answer **explains** the characteristic of the muscle fibre type clearly. It then goes on to expand the answer using a **specific** sports example. It uses **therefore** and **because** to link the answer together. Ensure you think carefully about the example you use – make sure it's appropriate in the context of the question.

## Compare and contrast

If a question asks you to compare and contrast the characteristics of different things (for example, the different muscle fibre types), then you need to make sure that you discuss the characteristics of both. Using words like WHEREAS or HOWEVER will help to link two parts of the sentence together to show that you are meeting the command word.

# Exam skills 3

In your exam, you will have some extended-answer questions to complete. These can be based on any topic covered in the learning aims.

## Answering extended-answer questions

Extended-answer questions will NOT have bullet points to guide you in your answer but each question will be phrased so that you can identify the required information for your response, if you know the subject area well.

- ✓ Take time to read the question carefully.
- ✓ Look for the key words in the question.
- ✓ Focus on those words that tell you what you need to write about.
- ✓ Do not just write bullet points!
- ✓ Do not simply repeat the words from the question without explaining them.

> It is a very good idea to do a quick plan before you write your answer to make sure you cover the key points.

## Key points to remember

For the extended-answer questions, unlike other types of question, you do not get a mark for every point you make. You are marked on your ability to:

- provide a full and balanced answer (which is why it is so important to identify the key words in a question)
- provide an answer that is well written and shows your full understanding of the topic in the question. Therefore, having identified the key words, it is essential that your response relates to all of them to achieve maximum marks.

Extended-answer questions can be based on any area of the unit. The extended-answer questions are designed to stretch you. A series of simple statements will not be enough for full marks.

---

Remember that in your extended-answer question it will not be sufficient to talk in general about a topic. For example, if you are asked to **analyse movement patterns** in a back flip in a gymnast's floor routine, you will need to **discuss** the **specific movement patterns** in that sporting action rather than simply discussing joint movements.

## Worked example

> The image shows a gymnast performing. There are several stages in completing the back flip. Analyse how joints and muscles interact to allow the gymnast to complete the back flip. **(8 marks)**

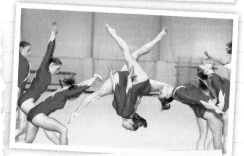

```
Prior to take-off the performer's hamstrings flex
the leg at the knee and the deltoids flex the
shoulder to aid momentum. Without this momentum it
is difficult to gain the necessary lift to perform
the flip.
During take-off, the gastrocnemius and soleus
plantar flex the ankle, the quadriceps extend
the leg at the knee to gain a powerful push
off, and the erector spinae extends the spine
to aid rotation. During flight, the hip flexors
and quadriceps flex the leg at the hip and the
abdominals and obliques flex the spine.
This allows the gymnast to form a tucked position,
without which it would be difficult to maintain the
backward momentum required to maintain speed and
rotation. Alongside this, the tibialis anterior
dorsiflexes the ankle to prepare for landing. After
landing, the quadriceps extend the leg at the knee
and the erector spinae extends the spine to allow
you to stand up straight.
```

If you are asked to analyse a topic remember these key points:

1. **Break the topic down** into smaller parts and clearly **identify each part**
2. **Explain each part in detail**
3. **Examine the relationship** between different factors, discuss how they **interact** with each other, and why this is important in the context of the sporting action.

# Answers

The following pages contain example answers to the 'Now try this' questions in Unit 1 of the Revision Guide. In many cases these are not the only correct answers.

## Learning aim A

### 1. Aerobic endurance

A triathlete needs good aerobic endurance because they have to complete long distances of swimming, cycling and then running without a break.

### 2. Muscular endurance

A 1500 m swimmer needs good muscular endurance because they need to provide enough energy to produce sustained movements at a moderate level over a long period of time. If they do not have good muscular endurance they will fatigue too quickly and their performance will decline.

### 3. Flexibility

| Performer | How is flexibility used in their activity? |
|---|---|
| Figure skater | To perform holds and positions with full extension, to score a higher mark for the routine. |
| Tennis player | To increase the power behind the serve by maximally rotating the arm at the shoulder. |
| Hurdler | Flexibility in the hip allows them to cross the barriers closely. |

### 4. Speed

$\dfrac{200}{24.5} = 8.16 \, \text{m/s}$

### 5. Muscular strength

| Performer | How is muscular strength used? |
|---|---|
| Sprinter | For maximum power out of the blocks. |
| Rugby player | For maximum impact in a tackle. |
| Gymnast | To gain maximum height and power when taking off from a vault. |

### 6. Agility

Basketball players need agility in order to move accurately and at speed with the ball so that they can place themselves in the correct position for a lay-up, while avoiding defending players.

### 7. Balance

Balance is important for a discus thrower to ensure that the athlete does not over rotate and place their foot over the edge of the throwing circle after the discus has been released.

### 8. Coordination

A netball player would use hand–eye coordination when catching a passed ball.

### 9. Power

A tennis player would need power to return the ball to the opponent at a fast speed. They also need power to make the ball go further and so harder for their opponent to reach.

### 10. Reaction time

If you are batting in cricket a good reaction time is important so that you make the correct decision quickly based on the type of ball that has been bowled at you. Wicket keepers must also have good reaction times in order to catch the ball.

### 11. The importance of fitness components for success in sport

During service when the ball needs to be released with one hand and hit by the racquet held in the other.

### 12. Exercise intensity: heart rate

$220 - 33 = 187$ bpm

### 13. Exercise intensity: the Borg (RPE) scale

The Borg (RPE) scale doesn't require the use of equipment so can be used anywhere.

### 14. Exercise intensity: training zones

$220 - 16 = 204$ bpm
$60 \times 204 \div 100 = 122$
$85 \times 204 \div 100 = 173$
The training zone would be between 122 and 173 bpm.

### 15. Basic principles of training

Aylin may start her training programme by working out once a week for 20 minutes, while her base level of fitness in swimming improves. After three weeks she should increase the number of times she trains to twice a week, which will help increase her aerobic endurance.

### 16. Additional principles of training 1

Suitable answers include:
Rowing machine – rowing
Exercise bike – triathlon
Treadmill – marathon running

### 17. Additional principles of training 2

If an athlete was doing a continuous training programme, they would need to ensure that they were working progressively harder over time in order to improve. For example, in their first session they could complete a 20-minute run at a 9 mph pace. Once this is no longer challenging they could increase the intensity by extending the length of the run, increasing the pace or increasing the number of times that they go running. If they repeat this pattern over time they will progressively overload their body.

### 18. Additional principles of training 3

(a) Working hours and a person's access to equipment.
(b) If a person spends a lot of time at work or works unsociable hours they are less likely to be able to attend classes or sport sessions that are held during the day and early evening. If a person lives in the countryside or in a more deprived area they may not have easy access to facilities such as gyms and swimming pools, and so their physical activity options would be reduced.

### 19. Additional principles of training 4

Adaptations are fitness improvements gained as a result of regular training. Reversibility is the opposite of adaptations and describes the process by which fitness improvements are lost as a result of not training.

### 20. Additional principles of training 5

Variation is important to ensure that performers remain motivated and interested in their training. It also helps to reduce the risk of injury by spreading the impact placed on specific body parts.

## Learning aim B

### 21. Circuit training

Station 3 – bowling at a target

### 22. Continuous training

$220 - 34 = 186$ bpm. 60% of $186 = 112$ bpm. 85% of $186 = 158$ bpm. Therefore, his continuous training zone would be between 112 and 158 bpm.

### 23. Fartlek training

A team player would focus on changing speeds rather than terrains as this is more similar to what they would experience in competition. For example, in football they would change pace while moving with the ball to outrun an opponent.

### 24. Interval training

Endurance athletes would have longer, moderate-intensity work periods whereas a power athlete would have short, high-intensity work periods.

### 25. Plyometric training

Plyometrics would be useful for triple jumpers as it would help them to develop explosive power and speed that could be used in their event. It also encourages them to use maximum force in a short period of time, which matches the requirement of their activity. (Accept any other suitable sport example.)

### 26. Speed training methods

In acceleration sprints, pace is gradually increased over time, whereas in hollow sprints, the pace is a flat-out sprint followed by a hollow period of jogging or walking.

### 27. Flexibility training

C  Active stretching

### 28. Weight training

Weight training reduces the risk of injury and allows for adaptations to training to occur.

### Learning aim C

### 29. Fitness testing: importance to sports performers and coaches

A  Consider changing the frequency, intensity, time or type of training as it currently might not be appropriate

### 30. Fitness testing: issues, validity and reliability

Ensure the time of day is the same, ensure it is conducted in the same environment, and ensure that the same warm-up routine is used.

### 31. Fitness tests: skinfold testing (body composition 1)

59 mm

### 32. Fitness tests: body mass index (body composition 2)

(a) Luke has a BMI of: $\frac{102}{1.8 \times 1.8} = 31$

(b) This BMI would classify him as obese. However, this test does not take into account muscle mass and it is likely that this is responsible for most of his weight. This means that he is probably not actually obese.

### 33. Fitness tests: bioelectrical impedance analysis (body composition 3)

A  Exercising before the test
D  Drinking before the test

### 34. Fitness tests: muscular endurance – abdominal

The test would not be reliable as conditions have changed.

### 35. Fitness tests: muscular endurance – upper body

A press-up test would not be appropriate because it does not use the abdominal muscles; it only uses the arms and upper body.

### 36. Fitness tests: speed – 35 m sprint test

Reliability may have been compromised as Fatima is running on a different surface in each test, meaning the results are not comparable: it may be harder to run on grass than a sports hall floor. As one test was outdoors, the weather may have affected her performance while this would have not have been an issue for the indoors test.

### 37. Fitness tests: multistage fitness test (MSFT) (aerobic endurance 1)

The football coach may choose to use the multistage test for a number of reasons. A large group can complete the test at the same time which means that the coach can test the whole team at once, which will save him time. The test is easy to set up, the coach only needs to measure the distance and mark this with two cones and then play a pre-recorded audio. The coach can choose to do the test either indoors or outdoors so he does not need to spend time finding a suitable venue. The test is a very useful way to measure a performer's ability; because players should not stop until they can no longer run, it will measure players up to their maximum aerobic capacity. This increases the test's validity.

However, the coach should be aware that the scoring of the test can be subjective as the players will choose when they are ready to stop running. This may not actually be when they can no longer continue. It is also easy for environmental factors to influence the result – if it is done outside it could be windy, which might mean the players can't run as fast as they might if indoors. But if the test is indoors, it may be too warm, which again may prevent players from running at their maximum rate. Equipment could be a problem as the test requires a specialist CD or recording; the coach will need to ensure he has the audio and a suitable device to play it on. Performers may find the test boring as it is very repetitive and this can affect their motivation and psychological state, which can impact on the results as they may give up on the test too early.

### 38. Fitness tests: forestry step test (aerobic endurance 2)

It is easy to administer and does not require any specialist equipment (like the MSFT CD).

### 39. Fitness tests: Illinois agility run test (agility)

It must be accurately measured each time to ensure that the test is reliable and results can be accurately compared with each other.

### 40. Fitness tests: vertical jump test (anaerobic power)

Any one from: he did not measure the height accurately; he did not complete the test in the same location or at the same time; he did not complete the test three times; it is likely his technique was not accurate as he did not warm up first.

### 41. Fitness tests: grip dynamometer (strength)

B  Weight training

### 42. Fitness tests: sit and reach test (flexibility)

A hurdler would score well on the sit and reach test because their lower back and hamstring flexibility are good. This is because they require flexibility in these muscles to assume the correct hurdling position and to pass closely over the hurdles. If they did not have this type of flexibility they would hit the hurdles more often and have to hurdle higher above the barrier, which would slow them down.

The following pages contain example answers to the 'Now try this' questions in Unit 7 of the Revision Guide. In many cases these are not the only correct answers.

## Learning aim A

### 46. Major voluntary muscles 1

The muscles found at the back of the upper legs are the **hamstrings**. Their role is **flexion** of the legs at the knees.

The muscles found at the front of the upper legs are the **quadriceps**. Their role is **extension** at the knees.

### 47. Major voluntary muscles 2

The pectorals are found at the front of the **chest** and are important when doing press-ups. The abdominals are found below the **pectorals** and allow flexion of the trunk. The obliques are found at the **side** of the waist and allow sideways flexion of the trunk.

### 48. Major voluntary muscles 3

**B** Soleus

**D** Gastrocnemius

### 49. Types of muscle

Voluntary muscles, also known as **skeletal** or striated muscles, are attached to the **skeleton**. Involuntary muscles, also known as smooth or **visceral** muscles, are found in the stomach, blood vessels and **intestines**. Cardiac muscle is only found in the **heart**.

### 50. Voluntary muscle movements

The **quadriceps** are the agonist when the striker extends his leg at the knee to strike the football and the **hamstrings** are the antagonist.

### 51. Antagonistic muscle pairs

Quadriceps and hamstrings.

### 52. Types of contraction

**1 B** When a muscle contracts but does not change in length

**2** Suitable answers include:
- During a football throw-in, the triceps have to contract concentrically to extend the arm.
- During a netball chest pass, the pectorals have to contract concentrically to push the ball forwards along with the triceps.
- During the Fosbury flop, the erector spinae has to contract concentrically to extend the back over the bar.

### 53. Slow twitch muscle fibres (type I)

Slow twitch muscle fibres are beneficial for endurance athletes because the muscle fibre characteristics match the demands of the events they compete in. Their events take place over a long distance, and slow twitch muscle fibres have the ability to produce force over a long period of time, are slow to fatigue and have a high aerobic capacity.

### 54. Fast twitch muscle fibres (type IIa)

**C** They are fairly resistant to fatigue

### 55. Fast twitch muscle fibres (type IIb)

**(a)** Any one from: produce the fastest contraction of the three muscle fibre types; produce the highest amounts of force, fatigue most quickly; produce explosive power.

**(b)** A sprinter in the 100 m needs to cover the distance in the quickest time possible so they need a high amount of type IIb muscle fibres. These allow their muscles to contract quickly and with the greatest force, allowing them to cover the distance in the quickest time.

### 56. Recruitment of muscle fibres with varied levels of muscular effort

When a long-distance runner starts a race they try to maintain a constant pace and so will recruit type 1 muscle fibres. If they find that they are falling towards the back of the group, they will need to increase their speed and will need to recruit a higher percentage of muscle fibres, and will start to use type IIa fibres. During the latter stages of the event (usually the last 200 m) they may need to increase their speed again to make sure they win their event. They will recruit type IIb muscle fibres in order to explosively pull ahead of the other athletes.

### 57. Bones of the skeleton

| Bone | Location |
| --- | --- |
| Femur | Largest bone in the body and leg |
| Radius | Largest bone in the forearm |
| Ulna | Smallest bone in the forearm |
| Clavicle | Smallest bone at the shoulder joint |
| Fibula | Smallest bone in the lower leg |
| Tibia | Largest bone in the lower leg |

### 58. Different types of bone

Flat bones, such as the sternum, protect internal organs like the heart. The sternum protects the heart by having a large surface area that covers the organ.

### 59. The axial and appendicular skeleton

**C** Pelvic girdle

### 60. Structure of the rib cage and vertebral column

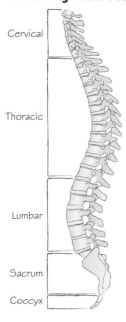

Cervical

Thoracic

Lumbar

Sacrum

Coccyx

### 61. Functions of the skeletal system 1

Muscles attach to bones via tendons. This is important because when the muscles contract they pull on the tendon so that movement can happen. During the long jump, if the muscles weren't attached to the bones the athlete would not be able to run or jump. This is true for all movements that occur.

### 62. Functions of the skeletal system 2

The four minerals that are stored in bones are: calcium, phosphorous, sodium and potassium.

### 63. Classifications of joints

**C** Synovial

### 64. Types of freely moveable joints

The carpometacarpal joint of the thumb is an example of a **saddle** joint.

The cervical vertebrae are an example of a **pivot** joint.

The knee joint is an example of a **hinge** joint.

### 65. Types of cartilage

Hyaline cartilage is found on the articulating surface of bones. It helps to act as a shock absorber to absorb the stress that is placed on the joint during movement. This is particularly important for athletes such as basketball players who are always jumping, because when they land there is a high amount of force that travels up through the legs. Having the hyaline cartilage on the ends of the bone helps protect the bone and joint from wear and tear.

### 66. Synovial joint structure

Tissues that join bone to bone and hold together bones that form a joint are called **ligaments**.

The fluid-filled sac between the tendon and the bone that helps to reduce friction is called the **bursa**.

### 67. Joint movements 1

The knee joint has gone from flexion to extension to allow the player to straighten his leg.

### 68. Joint movements 2

**Adduction** is the movement of a limb towards the midline of the body.

### 69. Joint movements 3

The ankle joint has gone from dorsiflexion to plantarflexion.

### 70. Joint movement and muscle group contractions related to sports performance

After the ball toss as part of the service, the knee goes from partial flexion through extension and the ankle goes from a slightly dorsiflexed position through plantarflexion. Both of these happen to aid the tennis player's technique. The quadriceps work concentrically and the hamstrings work eccentrically to allow the knee to move from flexion through to extension. The gastrocnemius works concentrically and the tibialis anterior works eccentrically to allow the ankle to go from a slightly dorsiflexed position to a plantarflexed position. On the racquet arm, the arm goes from a flexed position to almost full extension after making contact with the ball. In order for this to happen, the triceps work concentrically and the biceps work eccentrically.

### 71. Structure of the heart

One mark awarded for each correct label. (Either location for the semi-lunar valve is correct.)

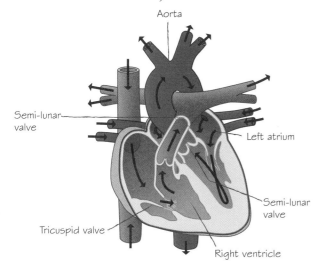

### 72. Types of blood vessels

Capillaries carry blood from arteries to veins by connecting **arterioles** and **venules**.

### 73. Functions of the cardiovascular system

If we cut ourselves, our blood **clots** to prevent further blood **loss** and **bacteria entering** the cut.

### 74. Functions of the cardiovascular system – thermoregulation

The body tries to maintain a constant internal temperature of 37°C. One of the ways the body does this is through vasoconstriction of blood vessels if the body detects a decrease in temperature. Arterioles under the surface of the skin narrow to prevent blood flowing to the surface of the skin. This stops heat from being lost through the skin, meaning blood will stay close to the core of the body (the brain and the organs).

### 75. Structure of the respiratory system

One mark awarded for each correct label.

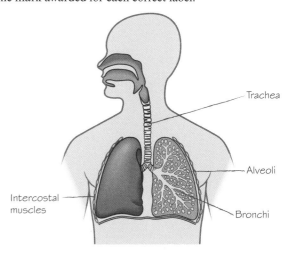

### 76. Functions of the respiratory system 1

During expiration, the internal intercostal muscles contract and bring the rib cage back down to its resting position. This forces the air out of the lungs.

### 77. Functions of the respiratory system 2

When we breathe in, the alveoli have a high concentration of oxygen and a low concentration of carbon dioxide, but the blood travelling to the lungs has a low concentration of oxygen and a high concentration of carbon dioxide. Gaseous exchange is when the oxygen moves from the alveoli into the blood and the carbon dioxide moves from the blood into the alveoli so that it can be expired.

### 78. Functions of the cardiorespiratory system

The **semi-lunar** valve opens, your **right ventricle** contracts and blood is forced into the **pulmonary artery** to travel to the lungs.

# Your own notes

# Your own notes

# Your own notes

# Your own notes

# Your own notes

# Your own notes

# Revision is more than just this Guide!

## You can get even more practice on each topic you revise with our corresponding Revision Workbook.

1-to-1 page match with this Revision Guide.

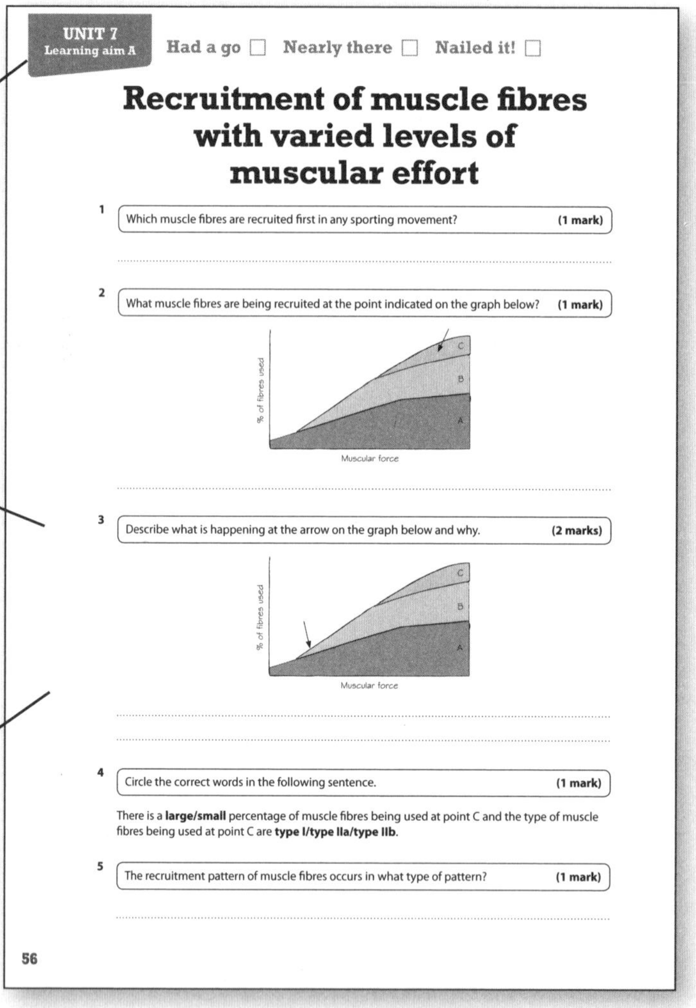

**UNIT 7**
Learning aim A

Had a go ☐   Nearly there ☐   Nailed it! ☐

### Recruitment of muscle fibres with varied levels of muscular effort

1  Which muscle fibres are recruited first in any sporting movement?   **(1 mark)**

2  What muscle fibres are being recruited at the point indicated on the graph below?   **(1 mark)**

3  Describe what is happening at the arrow on the graph below and why.   **(2 marks)**

4  Circle the correct words in the following sentence.   **(1 mark)**

There is a **large/small** percentage of muscle fibres being used at point C and the type of muscle fibres being used at point C are **type I/type IIa/type IIb**.

5  The recruitment pattern of muscle fibres occurs in what type of pattern?   **(1 mark)**

56

Guided questions help build your confidence.

Questions get you ready for your assessment test.

Hints will help you prepare for this topic in your assessment test.

Get ready for the test by completing our practice assessment test.

Sample page from Revise BTEC Sport, Revision Workbook

## Check out the matching Revision Workbook

Revise BTEC First in **Sport** Revision Workbook

978 1 4469 0671 2

THE REVISE BTEC SERIES FROM PEARSON

www.pearsonschools.co.uk/revise